To Mari
Irwin, ...
lady and precious.
friend .

Deborah C. Parsons

march, 2022

Talking Out of Both Sides of My Mouth

A Stroke Memoir

By

DEBORAH C. PARSONS

with Jerry A. Martin, Ph.D.

Dedication

To Jerry
and
Brooks/Genesis Rehabilitation Hospital

Introduction

I have written this book for anyone who has been unfortunate enough to experience a stroke, either first hand, or by a friend or family member. I have also written it in thanks to my fellow therapists and the physicians at Genesis/Memorial. My memoir is written from two points of view: one as a therapist, and one as a patient. This is why I am *talking out of both sides of my mouth.*

The field of rehabilitation medicine has evolved and progressed tremendously since 1995, when I experienced my stroke. Research continues to progress in diagnostic, as well as treatment areas, for both ischemic and hemorrhagic stroke.

Brooks Rehabilitation Hospital (formerly Memorial Regional Rehabilitation Hospital and Genesis Rehabilitation Hospital) in Jacksonville has a 50 year history of innovative services in healthcare and rehabilitation starting in 1969 with Memorial Hospital of Jacksonville. To learn about Brooks go to *https://brooksrehab.org*

The value and importance of a strong rehabilitation program cannot be over stressed. I was extremely fortunate to not only have the necessary health insurance for rehabilitation, but also access to the best possible rehabilitation hospital available. I was also fortunate to have the experience of working at Genesis, currently Brooks Rehabilitation Hospital. It was a wonderful place to work and it gave me a strong foundation for my recovery. According to The American Stroke Association, many people do not have access to sufficient rehabilitation services. This is very detrimental to the recovery of independence after an injury or stroke. Thank you for allowing me to share my story with you. I hope you will learn something that you did not know about the subject of stroke and the rehabilitation process.

Forward

Jerry A. Martin, Ph.D.

I am overjoyed that the love of my life has completed and published *Talking Out of Both Sides of My Mouth*. Due to the consequences of her stroke, this has taken over 25 long years. I am extremely proud of her for working such a long and hard time to finally finish her book. With her cognitive deficits, especially executive functioning, she was only able to work on the book for much briefer and less continuous periods of time than most writers. I believe that her process of writing was somewhat similar to making a list of some sort, for it has helped her to remember past events and, thus, overcome some of the memory problems that resulted from her stroke.

The title of her book applies to me, as well as her. This is true because I have a Ph.D. in psychology and during my career I have worked in two different rehabilitation settings. One would think that would have prepared me to face the problems and issues Deborah had when she was discharged from her rehabilitation hospital; however, working with someone with cognitive issues in a work setting is totally different from living full time with someone who has those problems. I do hope that I have been of help to Deborah in writing this book. She realized that she needed feedback, as well as editing of her writing throughout the years. I was happy and honored to provide that.

In the past, when I had been working, I had co-authored a text-book, written chapters for several edited books, served as an editor of a scientific journal, reviewed and edited several textbooks before they were published, and reviewed edited manuscripts submitted for publication in scientific journals. None of this prepared me for reviewing and editing Deborah's book. It was much too personal and I found it a challenge to change or edit what she had written. I also decided that I would not press her to spend time working on her writing and completing this book. She did not need added pressure from me considering all the pressure she had adjusting to her stroke. I felt that she needed to work on her own time schedule as best she could manage with her cognitive issues. Thus, she often went many months without spending any time writing and, in the end, it has taken over 25 years for her to complete her book. During that time she frequently revised parts of all of the chapters based on my input, input from her friends, and on her own decisions. While one major downside of the COVID-19 pandemic has been that Deborah and I have been "homebound" and less socially involved with friends and outside activities. Perhaps this time alone together did enable us to work together to finally complete *Talking Out of Both Sides of My Mouth*.

As I have said, I am very proud of Deborah for her considerable effort in finally publishing this book. I sincerely hope that you will find her book as interesting and enjoyable to read as I have.

Contents

Chapter 1—TGIF

At 8 a.m. on Friday March 24, 1995 at Genesis Rehabilitation Hospital, where I had been working as a cognitive rehabilitation therapist for about five years, I greeted 6 patients for a group therapy session. The purpose of the group was to assess the patients' orientation to person, place, time, and situation, as well as primary behaviors that might be the result of their injuries or indicators of the stage of their recovery. The group was an interesting mix of men and women that, in addition to stroke and brain surgery, were recovering from traumatic brain injuries of one kind or another.

Along with responsibility for the group, I had a caseload of 6 patients for individual sessions as well. I had two additional patients for a coma stimulation protocol. I would see three of the patients from the group for individual sessions later in the day. The other three would see a different cognitive rehabilitation therapist. During the group session I asked each person to tell me the day and date, including the year, as well as where they were and why. In addition, I asked a few general information questions such as who is the current president, what is the capital of Florida and other similar questions. In order to assess each person's progress, another therapist would take notes to include not only the answer each person gave, but also what behaviors they exhibited that might indicate a particular level of improvement or an issue to address in individual therapy. Because each person was wheelchair dependent, at the end of the session a courier came to take each person away and deliver them to another therapy elsewhere in Genesis. Each patient had a full schedule of therapies in addition to cognitive rehabilitation therapy, including physical therapy, occupational therapy, and speech therapy. They might also have biofeedback therapy.

At 8:30 a.m. after the therapy session ended, I went to my office to get my coma stimulation protocol kit to work with my patient that was just beginning to emerge from his coma of two weeks. Although he was no longer intubated, he was not yet fully alert. My kit contained items for stimulation of visual, auditory, olfactory and tactile senses. My kit also included my checklist and rating scale to document his responses to my administration of stimulation. After my session with this man I returned to my office to begin seeing patients for individual sessions.

At 3:00 p.m. I returned to the same group therapy room to work with another group of patients also recovering from brain injuries, but further along in their recovery. Unlike the morning group, the afternoon therapy focus was learning and memory. The goal of the therapy was to teach memory techniques and assess the ability of the patient to learn new information and put it into practice. The session lasted one hour, so at about 4:00 p.m., I said goodbye to them and watched as a courier escorted each person away.

After the patients were gone and my paperwork was completed, it was time to leave. I walked to my office to retrieve my purse and canvas bag of workout clothes, then locked the door and began walking toward the elevator. Walking down the hall I met a fellow therapist. She dramatically ran the back of her hand across her forehead and gave a simulation of shaking sweat from her hand, then she smiled and said, "Man what a week, T G I F!" I had to agree with her that the week had seemed longer than usual due to the high patient census.

As we stepped into the waiting elevator she said, "I don't know about you, but I'm wiped out." Then she looked at my bag and said, "Don't tell me you're going to step class." I said, "Hey, got to keep my schedule." Then she asked, "How can you possibly have the energy after today?" Then she added, "So, that's your secret for staying thin." I replied, "Oh, that's genetic, besides, working out doesn't make people short." She laughed and said, "Oh, right." Then I began shaking my finger toward her and added, "Shame on you, you know exercise is about staying healthy." Then I added, "Plus, I'm not getting any younger." She smiled and said, "I hear that." She asked me about my commitment to exercising, so I explained to her that aerobics had been a regular part of my life for more than ten years and how glad I was to be able to access HEART (Health Education and Rehabilitation Training), the health club associated with

Genesis. The fact that it was located very near the hospital made it nearly impossible to make excuses not to go. She asked me, "Are you going to TPC?" She was referring to the Tournament Players Club golf tournament. I answered, "Yes, and I hope the prediction for good weather turns out to be true." We talked a little more sharing anecdotes about some of our patients. Then as we parted and went our separate ways we both said, "See you on Monday."

After the aerobics class I drove home in anticipation of the next day's events feeling invigorated by the workout. As usual, I looked forward to attending the golf tournament. It was an event that had become a tradition for Jerry (my significant other of nearly ten years) and me. Similarly, it had become a tradition on Friday nights that we plan an Italian dinner centered on whatever wine we decided to drink. We would usually plan to prepare some Italian dish, either traditional pasta or sometimes a nontraditional dish. While the "Three Tenors" played on the stereo, I danced around the kitchen with a wooden spoon "conducting" dinner preparations. That evening our plans were to have our "Italian" night with an alternative to pasta with the customary red wine, a particularly good 1990 Chianti Classico.

We drank the wine with our dinner, then enjoyed our allotted one night of TV. Our guilty pleasure, "The X Files," was still being shown on Friday nights at that time. After the program, we went to bed. Not long afterward, I got up to go to the bathroom. I had no trouble walking or taking care of my business there. My speech was clear and normal as was my vision. After I was back in bed, Jerry asked, "How's your headache? I said, "I'm fine." Although I'd had a slight headache when I got into bed earlier, by the time I got back to bed it was gone. We both concluded that my headache was the result of my usual sinus problems being aggravated by the wine. It was not uncommon for either of us to have that experience.

I don't do early mornings. Aside from work, only a few things inspire me to rise early, especially on a weekend, TPC was one of those things. Because we had planned to go to the TPC golf tournament the next day (Saturday), we had also planned to go out to breakfast before going on to the golf course. Parking for TPC is always a challenge, so we had planned to get going early. Jerry was up before me, but that was typical. Still, after some time I had not followed him into the kitchen for coffee, so he decided to see if I was up. After seeing that I was still in bed he began trying to wake me. When his continued efforts failed to bring results, he became concerned. When I finally opened my eyes he was saying "Come on, we need to get going if we want to find a place to park. I thought you wanted to go to this thing." Then he said, "I guess you must have had more wine than we thought."

I was moving somewhat slowly and with a slight degree of difficulty, but since I didn't have any typical hangover symptoms nothing seemed out of the ordinary. I made my way to the toilet without difficulty but when I sat down I slid sideways into the wall on my left side. I thought that was strange, but I just assumed that in my groggy state that I had made some kind of misjudgment. It took some maneuvering to get out of the bathroom, but when I did I decided to go after Jerry to tell him that maybe something was wrong. As I walked out of the bedroom, he was just going down the hall to the door leading to the garage to collect our usual golf tournament gear. Before I could get to him, I fell sideways into the wall. He looked at me and said, "You're having a stroke, we're going to the hospital." I think I told him he was wrong and turned to go back to the bedroom intending to shower and get dressed. I was able to walk so it did not seem reasonable that a stroke was happening. Still, he followed me down the hall. When he caught up to me he maneuvered me to the closest mirror and said, "Look at your face and your arm." I was looking in the mirror trying to figure out what he was talking about. Then he said, "Okay, give me your left hand." It felt thick and heavy, and it was difficult to move. Then he said, "See, you're having a stroke, we need to get to the hospital." I said, "I can't go naked." I was wearing only my bathrobe. He said, "I guess you'll have to trust me then, I'll help you put on something easy." I asked, "What about my hair?" He said, "I don't think anyone is going to care about that, you've got bigger problems."

Knowing what an ordeal it might be in the emergency room made it a less than pleasant thought. Having worked with stroke patients as a therapist, I knew that if I were having a stroke, my life would be taking a serious turn for the worse. In addition, the hospital associated with my health insurance plan happened to be the one where I worked. It was especially difficult to accept the thought that people who might know me and/ or know my position in the hospital would see me. It was even more difficult to admit that I needed to go there at all. Those worries had to be set aside. I decided that they would probably find nothing wrong, send me home and we would go to TPC. We quickly got into the car and headed out to the hospital.

Since we lived in Ponte Vedra Beach, we had to drive some distance to get to the hospital. It was necessary to cross the St. John's River, affectionately referred to as "the ditch" by some of the local beach dwellers. The trip from our house to the hospital was one that I had driven every working day for almost five years. The view of dark green water and patches of reeds and grass and birds had always been a pleasant sight, but that day's drive is a blur in my memory.

After arriving at the hospital, Jerry parked the car near the emergency room (ER) entrance. By that time, I was unable to walk. My left leg seemed to be glued to the floor boards and my left arm stuck to my side. Trying to drag one half of the body with only the aide of the opposite side is an extremely difficult task. After trying to help me out of the car, Jerry decided to go for help. He said, "Wait here, I'll be right back." I said, "I don't think I'll be going anywhere just now." When he came back he was pushing a wheelchair and someone from the ER was walking with him. Together they got me into the chair with only a minor amount of difficulty. He kept joking about it being lucky that I didn't weigh too much. I, on the other hand, kept thinking that I was a lead weight. Every move was a tremendous effort leaving me feeling exhausted.

When we got into the ER, a nurse escorted us to an examination area and I was helped to sit on an exam chaise with a curtain pulled around it for privacy. Jerry stood next to me propping me up on my left side to keep me from falling. Working as a cognitive rehabilitation therapist presented very few occasions to pass by the ER, and in general, no reason to enter there. Still, the glare of the lights and sounds of voices and clattering of machinery or equipment, squeaking shoes and the smell of antiseptic seemed oddly familiar. The nurse left us there to wait for a physician. Jerry looked around and asked, "See anybody you know?" I said, "It's Saturday remember, we therapists get weekends off." After a few minutes, the same nurse came to check on us and she asked, "How are you doing here?" Jerry said, "Fine, I think. But she's too calm." It did seem that I was calm and unworried. Although I did have some concerns, my feelings seemed muted and still, almost numb. A loss of facial expression did not improve matters.

In a relatively short time a doctor came to see me. He pulled back the curtain that surrounded us and asked the nurse who was standing there, "What did you bring me?" He was very soft-spoken, asking the question as if he had been waiting for something. The nurse looked at him and said in an equally soft voice, "Stroke." It took only a minute for him to decide that a more complete evaluation would be needed to determine exactly what was happening. The emergency room doctor called my family practitioner, in accordance with the rules of my health insurance plan. After he made his assessment, it was obvious that a neurologist would be needed. Having never needed the services of a neurologist, the only ones known to me were those from work. The ER doctor asked me whom I would like to see. I had to make a decision but it wasn't a pleasant thought that a doctor I had worked with would suddenly become my doctor, especially given the situation. At the same time I began to realize that this would be the first of many, as yet to been seen, difficult decisions to be made. The ER doctor gave me a choice of two names. One I knew through work, the other I had only heard of in passing or read in some patient's report. In the end I decided on the more familiar doctor from work because I knew him to be good with people and a very contentious physician.

The gravity of the situation was beginning to set in. After reaching a decision, my choice of neurologist happened to be "on call" that day so he was called to make an evaluation. It seemed that he came to the hospital surprisingly fast. To Jerry it seemed that it was a very long wait. The neurologist made his initial assessment then ordered a CAT scan (computerized axial tomography). This is a process that uses a computer to produce cross sectional views from x-ray pictures. The CAT scan may also be used to investigate other areas of the body.

The CAT scan showed that there was something which needed more investigation. He said that a better picture of my brain would be needed to establish exactly what it was. He ordered an MRI (electromagnetic resonance imaging) for a better look. While there had been no occasion to see an MRI in progress during my time as a therapist, I had often read, with curiosity, about the procedure in reports about patients. It was not necessarily something I wanted to experience firsthand, yet there I was in the "long tube" that many of my patients had talked about. An MRI is a process that involves magnetism and radio waves and a computer to map body structures. The patient's descriptions had been quite accurate, and it was just as strange and loud as they had said. While there is no physical pain involved, it can be an unpleasant test. The imaging process creates sounds similar to a dull, thudding succession of hammering. The impression you get when you see the machine is its enclosed nature. Although it is not particularly small, it appears small from the outside, as well as the inside. In addition to being inside this metal cylinder, it is necessary to maintain complete stillness. Although I was able to see light past my feet, the enclosure was somewhat bothersome. It was also very difficult to remain perfectly still. Being inside this machine made it very easy to understand why a person with claustrophobia might not be able to tolerate the experience. To accomplish all this testing, someone pushed me in a wheelchair or on a gurney from place to place with surprising efficiency.

Later, the neurologist came to explain what the scans indicated. He told us that it was definitely a stroke. Specifically, there was a large right middle cerebral artery territory infarct (total blockage). I had already suspected that it would be a block or other problem somewhere in the right hemisphere since my left side was being affected. When I heard him say "middle cerebral artery" I knew that it was not good. Yet, I could not fully appreciate the seriousness of the problem until much later when the neurologist showed me the MRI pictures. There was no oxygen going to any part of the right hemisphere of my brain. That would turn out to more disastrous than I could have imagined.

After hearing his explanation of the problem, I understood why the early morning events had been unclear. The right hemisphere, controls physical functions on the left side of the body as well as the ability to recognize problems or discrepancies in various aspects of the body and/ or mental activity (awareness). Thus, my poor stability and physical features could not be interpreted as anything unusual. Looking at myself in the mirror showed no obvious problems. Whatever I saw evoked a "so what" response. It was as if the problem simply wasn't there. The lack of oxygenated blood in the right side of my brain caused the awareness system to cease function. Due to that fact, I was incapable of recognizing any physical abnormalities. When the awareness system of the brain doesn't function, there is no way to perceive a problem in the body. That is, until there is a need to use the side that is not working.

Given the test results, it was necessary to be admitted to the hospital's ICU (Intensive Care Unit). That seemed, to me, to be a bit of an overreaction at the time. The idea that my body was being affected by a loss of brain function was not totally real yet. There had been no emergency room drama with heroic efforts to maintain my life. I had not fallen or lost consciousness. Still, stroke situations are unpredictable; people sometimes die within hours or days of the onset of a stroke, depending upon many variables. With my clinical knowledge, I knew that admission to ICU was the normal procedure. It was, after all, a serious problem. At that time it was difficult to fully appreciate the seriousness. In addition, any previous experiences with hospital rooms involved work with patients destined for the rehabilitation unit of the hospital.

Being admitted into such a room created a very strange experience. I was suddenly in "patient" status rather than "therapist" status. The previous day I had worn a silk blouse with a linen skirt as well as heels and stockings. Now my clothes were replaced by the open in the back gown of hospital fame. The nurses worked to find the smallest pair of textured foot socks they could, but the smallest size was quite large on my child size feet. Although a kind nurse provided me with a second gown to wear facing forward to cover the rear, I very much wanted to get back into my normal clothes and leave. I was feeling very tired and suddenly very old. In addition to my new wardrobe, I had a variety of tubes and instruments attached to me and I was extremely tired. It was not only unpleasant, but emotionally unsettling to be out of my clothes and shoes.

My memories of the remainder of that Saturday are "fuzzy." Some of the tests and events of Sunday are stuck in my memory as being on Saturday. Regardless, there was more to follow after admission. The remainder of that Saturday was spent taking care of details, checking vital functions, medications, blood tests, etc. Sunday brought a new set of activities. Early Sunday morning a nurse came to make an assessment of my orientation to person, place, and time. This was so strange since on Friday I had been asking people these same questions. "What day is it?" Then there was, "Do you know where you are and why you are here?" It took a minute for me to collect my thoughts enough to come up with the correct day and date. Then came, "Where are you?" as well as "why you are here?" My immediate answer was, "Genesis," but after a quick look at the room I said, "No, wait, this is Memorial Medical Center." It seemed to me that my impression of the sequence of events that had brought me to the hospital was not quite accurate, but my knowledge of person, place, and time and situation was correct according to the nurse.

Later, the neurologist came to explain that yet another test would be needed to investigate more closely what might have happened in my brain and possibly why. The test he ordered in another effort to find the cause of my stroke was a cerebral angiogram. This complex and delicate procedure involves having a catheter inserted into an artery in the groin or in some cases the carotid arteries in the neck; the catheter is threaded through the artery to the base of the brain. Once there, dye is injected through the catheter in order to obtain clearly defined pictures of the arteries in the brain using the MRI again. It was another test familiar to me from my work-related reading. From the descriptions in surgical reports that I had read, it seemed to be a somewhat risky procedure, this could be especially true when the carotid arteries are the source of the problem. There is the risk that the catheter might dislodge another clot and send it into the bloodstream to end up in some other area of the brain and cause further damage or even death. I had previously thought that I might not want to have such a procedure. At the time there was very little choice. After "mild sedation" with Fentanyl (a drug I like to call "You won't remember"), along with a local anesthetic, the procedure was completed.

After the neurologist had reviewed the results of the test with the cardiologist, he came to discuss the results with Jerry and me. He told us that the angiogram indicated that an embolism (blood clot) had "probably" caused the stroke. He later explained that making a definitive distinction between a thrombotic (stationary) clot and an embolemic (moving) clot can be difficult.

Strokes come in two varieties: infarcts (blockage) and hemorrhage (bleeding). Infarcts generally have two basic causes, stationary and embolic clotting. A stationary infarct occurs when an artery becomes clogged due to a buildup of fatty material (cholesterol), also known as plaquing, in the artery. An embolic infarct occurs when a clot forms somewhere in the body and travels through the arterial system into the brain and becomes lodged in an artery that may be weakened or has narrowed as a result of cholesterol buildup or in a naturally narrow branch of a main artery. A hemorrhage occurs when a blood vessel ruptures due to excessive pressure on a weakened blood vessel or artery. Other causes are ruptures of aneurysms or AVM's (arteriovenous malformations). An aneurysm is the result of the wall of a blood vessel or artery stretching away creating a balloon shape. If the aneurysm ruptures, blood will spill into the brain cavity rather than reach its destination. An AVM is the result of twisted or bent blood vessels or arteries. These twists or bends may cause high blood flow and elevated pressure on the vessel that may, in turn, cause it to swell and burst.

Since an embolism was suspected as the source of my stroke, the neurologist ordered treatment with the anticoagulant, Heparin. Heparin and other drugs may be used to prevent the blood from making clots. These drugs are commonly referred to as blood thinners. Certain properties of the blood are altered by anticoagulants. In some cases, this can lead to serious negative side effects. In order to maintain a therapeutic drug level and reduce the chances of side effects, a continuous monitoring of the anticoagulant levels would be necessary. Therefore, a double channel IV catheter was inserted into my arm. This method enabled the nurses to take blood samples without interrupting the flow of medication. I hate needles so this was good because it made it unnecessary to have blood samples taken directly from my arm with a needle on each separate occasion.

I was an otherwise healthy and relatively young person (I had just turned forty-one the previous December). Also, the angiogram showed that my veins and arteries were in good shape. That left the question about a possible origin for the clot unresolved. In many cases the heart or lungs may be the origin; therefore, a look at those areas was necessary. A test used to further investigate this question was a transesophageal echo-cardiogram (TEEG). This test is accomplished by putting a long tube fitted with a transducer down the person's throat to obtain an ultrasound picture of the heart and its surrounding areas including the lungs. This test allows a close examination of the chambers of the heart including the arteries leading into and away from the heart. It is important to see if there are any abnormalities or an original clot formation that might be the source of the clot in the brain, a kind of parent clot.

I do not recall this test because it requires total relaxation. This was provided by a combination of Demerol and Versed along with some local anesthetic for the throat. In spite of the anesthetic, my throat was sore for the remainder of that week. All of these tests showed that everything in the areas tested was normal. According to the cardiology report, there was "no identifiable cardiac or aortic source for embolus." My heart was normal; my arteries, were, according to the cardiologist's report; "without plaquing" (cholesterol buildup), and with normal flow. My neurologist told me that I had a very good vascular system and that my arteries, heart, and lungs did not appear to be the source of the problem. It was comforting to know that I had a healthy vascular system but it made me wonder what could possibly have caused the stroke.

While the neurologist was talking to us, it occurred to me that I probably still appeared to be fairly calm. I was actually very scared and upset. The problem was that the stroke had affected my emotional reaction system both internally and externally. Although I had many concerns and fears, emotional reactions could not be projected. The technical term is "blunted affect." The outward expression (affect) becomes flat, giving the appearance of no expression at all. This also causes monotone speech. Much later, a close friend suggested that perhaps my seemingly calm reaction was not totally a result of the stroke but perhaps an exaggeration of my already strong resistance to breaking down under stress. That might or might not have been a factor at the time. If so, it was only a factor, not the cause. A loss of right hemisphere brain function was the direct cause. This aspect of injury to the right hemisphere had previously been a subject of my studies. It was also something exhibited by many people during the course of my work as a therapist. Having this knowledge was useful and frightening at the same time.

Even though all the tests showed no physical source for a clot in my heart, arteries, or other places, some physicians I have seen since my stroke have found this difficult to believe. This is natural because many strokes from embolisms generally originate in some part of the vascular system, particularly the heart or carotid arteries. Heart disease and stroke are very closely associated. Even so, it isn't always possible to find a source. Something had certainly happened, whether an obvious source was or was not found. That doesn't necessarily mean there is no cause. It is only that the cause could not be determined. In fact, in many cases of stroke, the cause is frequently labeled as "of undetermined origin."

All these tests were exhausting, and I worried that some new test might be ordered. Being pushed and pulled, lifted and carried, and otherwise aided for locomotion was extremely trying. Easy exhaustion was another effect of a stroke that academic study could not possibly explain. My familiarity with the immediate effects and future implications of a stroke came from my work as a therapist, as well as academic study. Those things made me familiar with various elements on an academic level. From exposure to other stroke survivors, the nature of how long and difficult recovery could be was also familiar. I was reminded of Martin Sheen's character in the film *Apocalypse Now*. He said, "I wanted a mission, and for my sins I got one." I didn't know about the sin part, but I wondered if my constant quest for knowledge and information was being rewarded in this way. It seemed that if this was a reward, that it was a dubious one that I could live my entire life without.

It was as if a rug or the floor had been suddenly pulled from under my feet sending me crashing. I would no longer be the person I had been only the day before. It was heartbreaking. I was stunned and weary. Like most people who find themselves being told that they are having a stroke, I wondered how this could happen and further, why was it happening? It was impossible to go home. It was impossible to do things independently. Walking was out of the question; therefore, going to the bathroom without help was not possible. That being the case, a urinary catheter was inserted. Additionally, I had only the use of my right hand. My left arm and hand did not move at all. Sensation (feeling) was there, but it couldn't move. There was no reflexive or purposeful movement. Instead, it felt extremely heavy. Like a lead weight, it hung at my side like a strange inanimate object. Although I could feel pain, even a severe burn would not have caused my arm to move. In addition, my face was distorted, my speech was slurred because only the right side of my face worked (I could not hear that it was slurred). In addition, weakness on the left side of my torso pulled me into a downward sideways slump.

All that aside, I began to think, and consequently worry, about work. It was clear that "see you on Monday" no longer applied to me. I worried about the possible impact of my absence on the other therapists. It made me unhappy to think about not being able to be there as usual, in addition to the reason. The remainder of that day, I dosed off and on trying to avoid negative thinking and worry. Fatigue and lethargy replaced my normal characteristics of activity and high energy. That made it somewhat easy to nap. The constant noise of people and equipment was difficult to ignore. By the end of the day I was settled into my room and eventually went to sleep.

Monday morning, looking around at the unfamiliar setting, I was disappointed to find that I was still in the hospital. It had been my hope that it was all a bad dream, I would wake up at home or wake up being able to go home. When I looked over the rail of the bed, I found myself looking at my supervisor. She was saying, "Good morning Deborah, how do you feel?" I thought that I should tell her that I felt pretty horrible, but the words wouldn't come. It seemed as if my life and spirit had been drained away. A weak "Good morning" was all I could manage.

Jerry had stayed with me most of the weekend, so he was standing behind her smiling and waving. My supervisor went on to assure me that there was no need for me to worry about my patients or my job. She had already taken care of those things. Jerry had called her, naturally, to let her know what had happened. Soon thereafter, the same questions about orientation to person, place, and time, as on Sunday, came from a nurse who quietly stepped into the room and stood nearby. After this initial activity of the morning, the day seemed to drag by very slowly.

Thankfully, Jerry had taken time off from work so that he could be there. By Tuesday, visitors, other than Jerry, doctors, nurses, and technicians, began to stop by to see me. In some ways it helped to see co-workers and friends, but it was also very hard. It was more than knowing my appearance was terrible. My stroke altered features combined with the lack of a shower and normal clothes made me feel like a slob. Although it was difficult to interpret their expressions, it often appeared that concern, worry, and sometimes shock was in their faces.

Monday and Tuesday passed slowly with very little change. Aside from being assisted to walk once in a while, there was little to be done. An important part of keeping physical systems working properly, and for safety, nurses and aides generally assist patients in some form of physical activity whenever possible. Yet, even with the assistance of a cane and a nurse, changes in my gait (manner of walking) caused by the stroke, made me sway and clump as I walked. When I looked down at my feet, they appeared to be turned in and downward giving the impression that I was walking on my arches. It reminded me of a seal's flippers. It was something that gave me a laugh, but it was a very brief laugh. Humor is at a premium in a hospital so you take what you can get. Nurses were sometimes unable to appreciate my odd attempts at humor and made little or no comment. As the week progressed, there was talk about the next step. It was necessary to determine whether rehabilitation would be appropriate. In some cases, an individual might be so severely impaired that rehabilitation would not be beneficial.

In order to make a determination regarding rehabilitation, it would be necessary to obtain evaluations from physical and speech therapists. That thought was discomforting because the therapists would most likely be coworkers from Genesis. The first evaluation was made by a young physical therapist whom I did not know very well; the next was made by a speech and language pathologist whom I knew quite well. It was impossible to decide which was worse. Both situations were uncomfortable for me and probably for each of them as well. By Wednesday, discharge became the topic of discussion. After reviewing the test results, the therapists and the neurologist agreed that rehabilitation would be appropriate. Since my medical condition was stable, the sooner rehabilitation started the better. The next decision was where rehabilitation would take place. The possible negative psychological effects of being treated by former co-workers were of considerable significance. Therefore, Jerry and I had talked with more than one doctor during the week about the appropriateness of a transfer to Genesis (the rehabilitation hospital) rather than another hospital away from Jacksonville. After weighing many pros and cons of the situation we came to the conclusion that Genesis was the best choice. Arrangements were made for the move to take place at the end of the week provided no new medical issues developed.

The decision to receive my rehabilitation at Genesis, although somewhat disconcerting, also seemed likely to be a positive thing. Over the years I had developed a tremendous respect for the professionalism and expertise of the people working alongside me. It was my forgone conclusion that the rehabilitation team would be excellent. Still, receiving therapy from friends and professional counterparts was difficult to imagine. The move to Genesis would come, but I didn't want to worry about it. I was far too tired.

I realized that I would soon make a trip across the walking bridge connecting Memorial Hospital and Genesis to begin the first phase of a very long recovery process. In addition, I could not know just how different it was to be a patient rather than a therapist. In preparation for the move, the neurologist ordered a gradual process of transitioning my anticoagulant from the IV form (Heparin) to the oral form (Coumadin). The standard procedure for reducing the IV form and starting the oral form is to reduce one and replace it with the other in equally small doses. It became time to think seriously about the saying, "I'll cross that bridge when I come to it." The walking bridge leading to the rehabilitation hospital was close enough to see from my window. Crossing that bridge would be very difficult. It would mean that the life I had known would be over, possibly forever, and a different life lay ahead. The uncertainty of the future was a prominent thought, while waiting for the transfer from ICU to the rehabilitation hospital. Again, I had no idea as to how different being a therapist was from being a patient. I had previously believed that I knew a great deal about strokes and the process of rehabilitation. Yet, I did not realize at that time that my knowledge was extremely limited.

Chapter 2—A Bridge!

Friday morning (March 31) a voice pulled me from my thick sleep. A nurse was saying, "It's time to wake up." She continued on with, "We'll be taking you over to Genesis soon and you need to eat something before you go." Not much later, after breakfast, a courier, who was very familiar from work, arrived with a wheelchair for the trip to the rehabilitation hospital. As he had been all week, Jerry was at the hospital after spending another difficult night trying to sleep in a chair that was in the room. Although it was difficult for him, it was important that he be there since he would be needed to assist in the complex process of a simultaneous discharge from one hospital and admission to another. The fact that we were not married had the potential to complicate that process.

The nurse and the courier worked together to position me into the wheelchair and, with Jerry following along, the courier began pushing the chair toward an elevator at the end of the hallway. The anticoagulant medication remained in IV form; the bag was hanging from a device known as an IV pole. The "pole" is made of metal and sits on a four wheel base. At the upper end is a set of inverted hooks where medication bags are hung for transport. In addition, the catheter had not been removed and the urine bag dangled on the back of the wheelchair. The urine bag would not be an issue for the courier, but he would be controlling a wheelchair and an IV pole simultaneously while getting from one hospital to the other. I remembered how difficult that task could be. As the pole wheels passed over a bump that sent it leaning precariously to one side, the courier deftly stepped sideways and caught it without interrupting the balance of the medication bag where it dangled from the top of the pole. Jerry commented to the young man, "You must have taken some course or something to learn how to do this kind of thing." The courier laughed and said "I've got this down after doing it for a couple of years." Smiling, he said, "I guess you could say it's on the job training." We both commented, "Practice makes perfect--- or something close to it."

A wheelchair is not a Toyota Camry. It felt like we were moving on a brick road instead of a smooth floor. As we exited the elevator on the second floor of the Memorial building on our way to the bridge, Jerry asked, jokingly, "Are you sure you know where you're going?" The courier replied, "Oh sure, I do this every day." He added, "The hospital is still working on changing a few things to make it easier to get around, thank goodness."

Working our way through the brightly lit halls, memories of the earliest days of my employment while rehabilitation was still a part of Memorial came back. Yet, those memories could not change a feeling of detachment from the surroundings. The hallways seemed as foreign as the first day that I had walked them. I had heard that before my employment at Memorial, there had been discussions among their board members about separating rehabilitation services from the hospital for various reasons. It was eventually decided that a new hospital would be built across the street on the nearest available property. It was decided that the new hospital would be called Genesis. It was a reference to new beginnings.

The design and appearance of the building was, and remains, a refreshing departure from a typical hospital environment. After moving into Genesis, the customary day-to-day activities took on a different air. The doctors, nurses, and other staff were always a strong, positive group of people. The atmosphere of care and concern they created would be evident in any environment. Giving them a fresh new environment added to their positive approach.

The most important thing for me was that this was not a show. Everything was very real rather than a pretty façade created to hide a lack of substance. It was real both physically and service-wise. Things were done for the comfort, care, and safety of patients. It was a place everyone felt good about. Having come to work for the hospital after previously working for a for profit rehabilitation company (not a hospital), my job was a relief. Any similarities with those two jobs ended with similar clinical staff and services. Genesis turned out to be the opposite of that experience for many reasons other than the few similarities. After exiting the last elevator on the second floor of Memorial, we continued on the path to the entrance of the bridge where we would leave Memorial and continue on into Genesis.

We continued on, moving closer and closer to the entrance to the rehabilitation hospital. Along the way it was easier to have negative thoughts rather than positive ones. It was disconcerting to imagine the possibility of seeing some doctor or therapist that I knew, or a patient that I had been working with up until the Friday of my stroke. It was difficult to imagine how it would make either of us feel. In any case, it was an unpleasant thought. In addition to those thoughts, knowing the many unusual aspects of my situation made it difficult to see resolutions for them. At that particular moment it was better not to think about those things. Jerry held my hand and said, "Try to relax." To that I replied, "Easier said than done."

Being a naturally positive person, I chose to think about the more immediate situation, and not worry about things yet to come. While the ramifications were vast, the rehabilitation hospital stay would not last forever. That was a very important thing to remember. In addition, it seemed obvious that my work experiences and personal strength would help in coping with whatever might be ahead. The doctors, nurses, other therapists, as well as patients had taught me many of the basic aspects of rehabilitation that would be beneficial to me. They had taught me a great deal more than they could know. Most importantly, the full support of a true partner and friend was involved. Still, accepting therapy and medical treatment from previous co-workers would be a supreme test. Here, Deborah the therapist, would be separated from Deborah, the patient. The entrance into Genesis loomed ahead like the entrance of a dark cave. The thought of entering Genesis as a patient was more bizarre than could be imagined. I did not want to go there in my condition. It seemed as if Rod Serlings' ghost might be found peeking around a corner someplace inviting us to enter "The Twilight Zone."

In spite of a few bumps and near collisions, we managed to make it to Genesis without losing the medication bag or pulling out the IV. As we arrived it was certain that crossing the threshold into Genesis would be very different from the last day that I had worked. Still, nothing could change the course of events from that point on. There was no choice but to face what might lie ahead. When we reached the point in the bridge where a security camera hangs from the ceiling, I made my customary wave to the unit secretary who watched the monitor in the nurse's station and I mouthed, "Hi." I've never known if she had seen me do that in the past, but I have always made the effort when walking in either direction across the bridge. After getting through the entrance to Genesis, leaving the sunlit bridge, the subdued lighting and hushed atmosphere seemed very strange rather than familiar.

After our arrival, the first order of business was to check in at the nursing station on the third floor which was the stroke unit. After completing a great deal of paperwork, we were taken to a room that was very different from my ICU room at Memorial. It was surprising to find that it was one of the larger rooms called "suites." The appearance of the room was another example of attention given to form along with function. All rooms at Genesis were basically large in order to give patients some space for their sometimes-lengthy stays. The suites had some added space.

Naturally, there is a finite amount of space in any building, but there was an effort made at Genesis to maximize the use of space as efficiently as possible. The room had a pleasant, hotel-like quality to it. The walls, like the other rooms in Genesis, were a soft peach. There were two small tables, and in the middle of the room, the bed. There was also a chair and a small sofa that were covered in a peach/teal print. For clothes, there was a large wardrobe with a television set into it, much like those found in hotels. On the adjacent wall to the wardrobe was a "vanity" table.

It was obvious that much thought had been put into the style of the room. At that point in time, there was no way to know how long my stay would be. It was nice to know that there would be some reasonable space to "live" in as long as it was necessary. The best feature of the room was a window. While the view over the parking lot wasn't exactly resort quality, it <u>was</u> a window.

Some former patients had joked with me about their rooms being a "home away from home." It was impossible to think about the room as home even for one day. My thoughts were about how much I missed my home. A more difficult thought would be when Jerry would leave for work. Because he had been away from work for so many days, he wanted to get back to it that afternoon. He could not be there throughout my entire stay at the rehabilitation hospital. It was a fact that was clear. Nonetheless, it was extremely unpleasant to think about.

I have always been a very independent person and generally comfortable about being on my own. Traveling out of town for educational conferences independently or staying at home while Jerry traveled was never a problem. Suddenly, it was difficult to think about being without him for even short periods of time. This separation would be an entirely new situation unlike any we had been through before. My loss of independence now extended beyond physical limits to the limits of being "taken care of." Additionally, it meant being watched over. It was like suddenly being dropped into a goldfish bowl in a room full of people. Each person in the room would be concerned for my safety and doubtful of my ability to do the same for myself.

Thankfully, Jerry was able to stay long enough to help get me settled in. It was difficult to see him leave, but I knew he would return the next day (Saturday). It became time to make a choice to either settle in for the rigors of therapy or mope around in self-pity. There were still so many difficult issues and details to be resolved. It meant there would be a lot of waiting for uncertain outcomes. In addition, it was obvious that a great deal of work remained before therapy activities could begin. Many aspects regarding therapy were yet to be decided. The initial sequence of events, however, would be fairly straightforward. Specific tests would be performed in order to construct a full therapy plan. After that, decisions regarding therapist and physician assignments had to be dealt with.

Because I had worked in the hospital, it would be important, as well as difficult, to avoid dual relationships (similar to conflict of interest) between people and myself with whom I might have worked very closely. Making testing and other treatment assignments would be a sensitive issue. Although allowances would be made for my input, final decisions would not be under my control because only so many therapists and time slots would be available. Availability would take precedence over other factors. One of the most difficult aspects of creating a therapy program is the schedule. A therapist is at the mercy of the level of occupancy of the hospital. Apart from that, it would be important that people that did, or did not, work with me not misunderstand the circumstances regarding therapy or other treatment assignments.

It would be particularly important, as well as tricky, to prevent anyone being offended by thinking that I might refuse to work with him or her. There was always a chance that someone would think that there was some personal objection on my part if they were not being assigned to my case. They might not recognize it as the blessing in disguise that it might be. There were no personal issues involved, and I didn't want anyone to think there were. This simply was not a common, everyday situation. Being an employee who had treated people recovering from strokes and other types of brain injuries was an unusual situation at the very least. Close working relationships, created by our interdisciplinary program style, with nearly every doctor, nurse and therapist in the brain injury and stroke programs further complicated the situation. Thinking about all of this was very tiring and stressful. Some of the things I had worried about were actually happening. Many former co-workers would see my thoroughly incapacitated state.

On Monday, my supervisor came to discuss what she considered to be some of the more pressing problems. In her position as a neuropsychologist (neuropsychology is the study of brain-behavior relationships), she would be involved in making decisions regarding many of the testing and therapy assignments. We talked about the dual relationship issue and explored a variety of solutions. One option was to move to some other facility. This was not an appealing idea because it would mean a geographical separation from Jerry. Being separated by hospital confinement would be bad enough. Thankfully, Jerry continued to visit each day after work. The time we had was very strained and difficult.

Constant fatigue and rules that prohibited leaving the building put further limits on us.

In rehabilitation hospitals, time constraints exist for completing evaluations, formulating therapy plans, and predicting lengths of stay. Given that, it would be necessary for the process to move along at a reasonable pace. I knew that it would be very few days before the initial phase of testing would start. While the physiatrist (physical medicine and rehabilitation specialist) had made an assessment of my physical problems, making an assessment of cognitive problems would require cognitive testing from a neuropsychologist (a neuropsychological evaluation). From there it would be possible to proceed to development of a rehabilitation plan.

The neuropsychological test, or more accurately, group of tests, had been an important reference tool for constructing treatment plans during my work as a cognitive rehabilitation therapist. My familiarity with the tests was academic rather than personal. Knowing that the evaluation would establish a foundation for a complete rehabilitation plan was a very intimidating thought.

The initial evaluation is not a complete battery of tests, but rather a set designed to evaluate specific brain functions based upon the area of the brain and the type of stroke that an individual might have experienced. That particular knowledge was not comforting. It was obvious that the tests would show numerous cognitive deficits created by my stroke. Problems that did not exist before the stroke would be revealed. A lengthy wait would have been preferable, but that would not be possible. The time would come all too soon.

In addition to the neuropsychological evaluation, each therapist would eventually conduct evaluations specific to their particular disciplines and use the neuropsychological evaluation as an additional reference. Using these tools they would construct a treatment plan designed to address each area of deficits, whether physical or cognitive, created by my stroke.

Besides finding therapists for therapy services, there was the challenge to decide the best way to deal with the initial evaluation. There were three possible choices of neuropsychologists, but each person was very familiar with me due to our close work relationships. After a great deal of discussion a decision was reached and the evaluation was scheduled for the Wednesday after my admission into Genesis.

It was mid-morning on Wednesday when the time came for the test; a courier pushed me in my wheelchair to a testing room. I was told that there would be a brief wait before the session could begin. In only a short time there would be activities for me to perform and questions for me to answer. In the meantime, it was just a matter of waiting. Jerry was included in the testing session in order to verify particular information.

Although I had been informed as to the identity of the tester, it was a surprise when she walked through the door. We shook hands, and she asked, "Are you ready for this?" I thought jumping out of a plane might be easier. It was not simply a matter of apprehension regarding the testing. The entire experience was very tiring. The pencil and paper activities seemed laborious to me and when she asked me questions, I felt more challenged than I expected.

Prior to the stroke, my strength and stamina had been good. Dedication to aerobic exercise over the years had been beneficial in both areas. An injury to the brain will usually reduce a person's stamina level. Due to the stroke, my typical characteristics of high energy, enthusiasm, and stamina were replaced by lethargy, fatigue, and apathy. This particular aspect of stroke is a difficult contradiction for every survivor as well as friends and family. In order to recover strength and stamina, physical activity must take place. The loss of previous levels of strength may reduce a person's desire to participate in therapy activities. Therapists or family members may mistake this for a lack of motivation when in fact the injury itself causes the problem. After the test was completed, it was possible to get a much needed rest in the afternoon. The heart and soul of rehabilitation is work, both physical and cognitive. Physical and cognitive exercises go hand in hand. The term "aggressive therapy" is not taken lightly. There is very little in the way of inactivity in a rehabilitation hospital.

Having reviewed the various test results, the neuropsychologist met with Jerry and me to explain that the neuropsychological evaluation revealed loss of cognitive function in areas such as attention and concentration, visual perception, facial and vocal affect (expression), as well as higher level critical thinking and organization skills. As it might be expected, this information was used to create a rehabilitation plan that would include occupational therapy, physical therapy, speech and language pathology, and biofeedback.

Physical and occupational therapies would naturally be included in the program to address the various physical disabilities created by the stroke. Once a physical therapist explained to me that the two therapies share common definitions as therapies to restore physical function and prevent disabilities through encouraging the return of range of motion and retraining ADL (activities of daily living) skills. To reach these goals, individual as well as group therapy sessions are included in many rehabilitation programs. Although I did not fully understand the work of the physical and occupational therapists, I always found it interesting to observe a patient of mine interacting with them. In my early days at Genesis, I was hesitant to query these therapists about their work, but I found them to be very open and easy to talk to about the activities that they provided for therapy. Now I would be the one interacting as a patient with those therapists. I had previously learned from some physical and occupational therapists that along with their shared definitions, physical and occupational therapies might sometimes share the misperception that they are purely physical in nature when in reality both therapies involve cognitive as well as physical activity. Physical activity is dependent upon cognitive activity.

Paralysis from brain injury is not the result of severed nerves in the limb or spine; it is an incomplete state of paralysis known as paresis. The brain is unable to communicate necessary information that would normally be delivered to specific areas of the body. In right hemisphere damage, the left side is unreachable. In left hemisphere damage, the right side is unreachable. The injured brain area has lost its connection to the parts of the body that it controls. The brain does not know that it isn't sending information to a limb because it doesn't recognize that the limb is there. The prevailing theory in rehabilitation has been that when physical function is disrupted due to an injury, the brain must become "recon-nected" to nonfunctioning areas. Further, since the nerve system of the body is intact, the brain can be "reconnected" to the affected areas through therapeutic activity. Directing activities to the affected area of the body stimulates the brain-body connection. There are many theories about how and why this is possible.

For therapeutic activities designed to improve cognitive and phys-ical functions, therapists require a variety of equipment and safe, com-fortable places for patients to perform exercises or practice various therapeutic tasks. While a physician in his or her office might perform some therapeutic applications of medication or certain types of muscle stimulation, the bulk of physical activity takes place in a therapy gym. Some therapies are conducted in private office spaces in order to reduce distraction and provide appropriate equipment or tools according to the type of therapy to suit an individual patient's needs. As a cognitive reha-bilitation therapist, my work had been accomplished within a private space where there were no interfering or competing activities.

The therapy gym at Genesis is typical of rehabilitation gyms any-where, bustling with activity and sounds created by patients and thera-pists interacting throughout the process of therapeutic activities, as well as a normal flow of assorted staff and visitors coming and going. As a therapist, visits to the therapy gym were generally related to gaining some firsthand information about the progress of a patient. It was always an active and dynamic place. Now, I would be going to the gym, not walking in my heels, but rather being pushed in a wheelchair. This was very unusual for me, as much as anyone else with a stroke.

Another part of a therapy program is speech and language pathol-ogy, most commonly referred to as simply "speech therapy." I was told by a speech and language pathologist that, like physical and occupational therapies, speech and language pathology is a complex issue. Communication is not limited to the act of speaking. The production of speech is one element of the complex process of verbal communication. Other elements involve the ability to use words in a functional manner (language). Word production alone is not sufficient. Vocalization has unique features apart from the appropriate use of words to communicate. There are various impairments of the speech organs and swallowing apparatus that are far too complex and lengthy for discussion here and beyond the scope of my knowledge.

Speech and language pathologists study the organs of speech, and the processes involved in communication along with their connections in the brain in order to understand not only the mechanics of speech, but the comprehensive elements of communication as well. They study what can happen when areas in the brain responsible for speech or language usage become damaged. When strokes are discussed, it is common to hear references to the inability to use language properly or having an inability to speak. The most common effect referred to is slurred speech. This is generally the result of inactive muscles on one side of the face. Language use may become impaired in ways other than the ability to speak or to speak clearly. Also, every speech or language problem does not occur in all strokes. I was fortunate to be spared the problems of any form of aphasia. I would have a very different language problem resulting from my right hemisphere damage.

From the speech pathologist I also learned that language use is divided into two main categories: receptive (input or understanding) and expressive (output). The functions of both receptive and expressive language are attributed to certain areas in the left hemisphere of the brain. Monitoring of language and expressiveness is attributed to areas of the right hemisphere. If a stroke or other injury affects areas of the left hemisphere where language usage is controlled, a loss of ability may occur in various ways dependent upon the severity and location of the injury. When an injury occurs in the area of receptive speech, understanding words may be impaired. This type of impairment is known as Wernicke's Aphasia (named after the German physician Carl Wernicke). If the injury affects the expressive area, the ability to use or produce words properly becomes impaired; the person knows what they want to say, but cannot say it. This is known as Broca's Aphasia (named after the French physician Paul Broca). Additionally, a condition known as apraxia may occur as the result of an injury. Apraxia is the inability to use objects properly. In any of these situations the ability to function in the speaking world is changed. Very suddenly a person may lose their ability to make sense of what is said to them or to make correct use of words to communicate their needs to others. Impairments may be auditory (hearing) or visual (written) or a combination of both. If injury occurs in the right hemisphere, the ability to monitor the way one speaks or how much may be impaired. Speech and language pathologists address these problems according to each individual's needs. Most human endeavor and interaction is based on communication in some form. Therefore, rehabilitation therapies in all disciplines address many common areas. Memory and learning, language use, logic, behavioral awareness and control, neglect of visual fields or limbs are just a few.

Well known for its use in pain management, but less common in stroke rehabilitation programs is biofeedback. The biofeedback therapist explained to me that biofeedback is a therapeutic method for teaching control of the autonomic system such as heart rate, blood pressure, skin temperature, and relaxation. This is accomplished through the use of monitoring devices and computer programs that give auditory and/or visual feedback to the individual when a goal is reached. By knowing what event produces a change, an individual tries to reproduce the event on command to achieve the desired results. The techniques can be especially useful in addressing problems such as blood pressure, heart rate, and anxiety. Aquatic therapy, also not widely available in rehabilitation hospitals, is another addition to rehabilitation programs at Genesis. Aquatic therapy involves using a pool to provide occupational and physical therapy exercises.

Every aspect of brain injury recovery, regardless of the injury's origin, requires vigorous activity. The physical aspects alone require immediate and sustained activity. Although a person may have been active and/or athletic prior to their injury, they will find every aspect of rehabilitation to be strenuous and difficult, regardless of their motivation. Being physically strong prior to an injury doesn't prevent rehabilitation activities from being tiring or difficult, but it may help to get recovery off to a good start. Another important aspect of getting a good start is to get a rehabilitation program started as early as possible. Given the ambitious program that was ahead of me, it was welcome to know that the program was scheduled to begin the following Monday.

Chapter 3—Work, Work, Work

Although every day presented challenges for basic activities such as getting out of bed or any normal morning task, the first day of my rehabilitation program was, perhaps, the most difficult. As usual, the lack of function on my left side made it seem as if I was tied down. More unpleasantly, it continued to be necessary to monitor my anticoagulant level on a daily basis. Since the double channel IV line had been removed, it became necessary to draw blood through a syringe. This was done first thing every morning.

On the positive side, Jerry arrived just after breakfast. He had come by to wish me luck on my first day of therapy before going to work. With assistance from both the nurse and Jerry, it was eventually possible to get out of bed. My complaints about the cold hospital environment had prompted Jerry to bring me an old soft flannel pajama set. One of my sisters would later name them "prison" pajamas. The flannel added a minor amount of difficulty with getting out of bed since the pants were long and the flannel dragged along the surface of the sheets.

Aside from the lack of function on the left side of my face, causing me to chew on the inside of my cheek and lower lip, my ability to eat independently was not affected. Thankfully, the catheter had also been removed along with the IV line. This was much to my relief in spite of the change in blood draw method. Soon after Jerry had arrived, an occupational therapist, whom I did not know well, came in to begin a therapy session for training and assistance in ADL's (activities of daily living). These activities include self-care such as hygiene, eating, dressing, and simple meal preparation. At first, the idea that a fellow therapist would assist me to dress or complete any other self-care task had been extremely unpleasant. Since we were not very familiar with each other, it was a little easier to greet her. The therapist smiled and said, "Let's get started." Getting started was not only unpleasant, it was extremely difficult. Clothing is not designed for single handedness. The everyday elements of dressing are normally easily accomplished without conscious efforts. After a stroke these activities become something requiring intense concentration with intentional, rather than automatic, behaviors. Pulling up pants, pulling down shirts, buttons, zippers, socks, and shoes take much more work than anyone would consider under normal circumstances. Dressing was no longer an easy automatic activity. Jewelry was not an issue since I would not be wearing any for therapy. Getting into a bra was impossible. In light of that fact, I sent Jerry on an errand to bring one of my one piece pullover style bras from home. Unfortunately, this too turned out to be just as impossible as pulling on a t-shirt. Fortunately, my lack of significant endowment had in general made me less concerned about a bra. Being in situations that did not require a polished professional appearance also made it less important to me. The cool temperature in the hospital made wearing a jacket a good idea. That served to help with the bra issue as well.

One very good thing was that it was possible to be independent in brushing my teeth. Flossing, on the other hand, was not simply accomplished. Although the therapist made an effort to teach me a one handed method for holding the floss, it turned out to be too difficult. When I explained to her that it was not acceptable for me to skip such an important part of oral hygiene, she suggested floss picks. Jerry bought some and it was then possible to floss. Although they were not optimal, they provided an effective temporary solution to the problem.

The therapy team assigned to my case worked together to create a program that included group, as well as individual therapy sessions. The first therapy after the ADL session in my room was an occupational therapy range of motion (ROM) group. Later in the day, a different occupational therapy session would be conducted on an individual basis. When the ADL session was over, it was time to move on to the next therapy. After the OT had gone, a courier arrived to transport me to the occupational therapy group session. Jerry said, "Okay, play times over." After assuring me that he would return to spend dinner time with me, he kissed me and said, "Good luck."

Both physical and occupational therapy sessions would take place in the therapy "gym" on the first floor. My room was on the third floor, which meant there would be many opportunities to see previous co-workers while moving from one therapy to the next. That was an unpleasant thought. Although it might be enjoyable to see those people, the idea that they would see me was not.

Generally speaking, I am not an anxious or nervous person. In fact, from the beginning of my life my nature has been one of optimism, as well as determination and what is often considered to be stubbornness. These attributes might be connected to my start as a barely 5 pound baby and transition into a petite, but hardy adult. I could be intimidated, but not easily. Anyone that tried intimidation on me would quickly recognize their mistake. On the other hand, thinking about the beginning of therapy, it was easy to imagine the worst. Normally such a situation would find me fully prepared to face whatever had caused my condition, ready to attack the problem head on. Instead, I was resigned to the control of a regimented system created by other people. There was a conflict between being ready to begin therapy, and a fear of beginning. Being in the wheelchair accentuated negative aspects of the situation.

As the courier pushed my wheelchair down the hall to the elevator, I said, "Now for the fun part!" She laughed as the elevator door opened and we were on our way to the first activity of the day. It was more intimidating than I had believed that it might be. Still, it was something easily reconcilable by the realization that it was necessary. If abilities were to be recovered, therapy was the best way to make it happen.

We arrived at a very familiar range of motion (ROM) group room just after 8 a.m. The therapist and nursing assistant moved each of the patients into a circle around a large table and helped everyone sit upright as well as it was possible. When everyone was ready, the session began. The activities consisted of using our functioning arms to facilitate movement in our nonfunctioning arms. Many activities involved moving the non-functioning arm in various motions and directions. It was obvious that the overall activity level of each patient in the group would not be returned for some time, but day-by-day improvement in tolerance for the group was encouraging to both patient and therapist alike. Just like me, every stroke patient showed the effects of physical problems preventing them from taking their usual care with grooming. Everyone expressed a change in self-image. In his book, My Year Off, Robert McCrum expressed the image he had of himself as "a beetle or cockroach without a leg flailing helplessly and covered in dirt, on the brink of extinction." As a therapist, I had often heard patients say that they felt "ugly." My concept of myself had changed from that of a cheerful, competent, well-groomed professional to that of a dowdy, lopsided, expressionless lobotomy subject. In addition to physical appearance, damage to the right hemisphere of my brain caused dysfunction in the system controlling facial expression and voice. My voice had become monotone. It was completely different from my usual voice and facial expression. It was no longer possible to communicate through vocal inflections or body language. This compounded the altered self-image I had developed. At some point, my mother and one of my sisters came to visit. Changes in both facial and vocal affect had a negative effect on them. The failure to show facial expression and speak normally gave the impression that their visit was nothing unique or even appreciated. The same misunderstanding seemed to effect Jerry as well.

To add to this new image, my naturally curly hair had become rather unruly. Unfortunately, it was overdue for a cut, and with only one hand to work with, keeping it properly groomed was impossible. Under normal circumstances, having long hair would be nothing more than inconvenient and time consuming. That was not the case in the hospital. To make matters worse, it was not possible to leave the hospital to get a haircut. That was particularly annoying since I considered it to be a matter of my mental health. As usual, Jerry is walking around singing "Help me Rhonda." This is what he does at home when I have put off a haircut for too long.

Fortunately, my hairdresser, Rhonda Felder, was not only a gifted stylist, but a great person as well. When Jerry explained the situation to her, she volunteered to provide a cut at the hospital. She said that she would, "take the haircut to Deborah." One afternoon, after therapies were over, she came to the hospital and created a style that would be easy to manage even with one hand. It was such a relief to have some control over something, especially something related to appearance.

After the ROM group, it was time to continue on for an individual physical therapy session. The therapy gym at Genesis was typical of rehabilitation gyms everywhere, bustling with activity and sounds created by patients and therapists interacting throughout the process of therapeutic activities, as well as a normal flow of assorted staff and visitors coming and going. As a therapist, visits to the therapy gym had generally been related to gaining some firsthand information about the progress of one of my patients.

The courier brought me to the first floor lobby area, where a number of other patients sat in wheelchairs waiting to be taken to their next scheduled therapy. I was left next to an elderly woman in a row of patients immediately facing a wall near the gym. After a few minutes she turned to me and asked, "When does the movie start?" I said, "I think someone will be here soon to take us to therapy." She replied, "We're not going to see the movie?" It seemed obvious that she was somewhat confused about the situation, so any further discussion might not be helpful. Fortunately, the courier arrived and began "driving" my wheelchair into the gym and stopped at a set of mats where a physical therapist, with whom I had often worked, was waiting. She greeted me with a warm smile and said, "Good morning Deborah." We didn't spend time with small talk. We had important business to attend to. Looking around the gym, there were other patients with strokes or other types of brain injuries going through the same process or already far into their sessions. Some were working through the strain and frustration with intense determination, while others railed against the therapist with anger and resistance. Some were simply too confused to fully participate.

My therapist began each session saying, "Let's get you out of the chair and onto the mat." She often made me laugh by saying, "Hop up here on the mat." The latter I would not be doing at all. The former I would be doing until it was no longer necessary. Getting from the wheelchair to the mat would not be simple. Numerous steps would be necessary in order to make the transfer. First, the brakes on the chair would need to be put in the locked position to prevent its rolling. Next, the footrests were moved out of the way in preparation for the transfer from chair to mat. This process may sound fairly simple, but it is in fact a very complex physical, as well as cognitive task. It was accomplished through a series of actions starting with holding onto the therapist with the functioning arm and then slowly standing on the functioning leg. With help from the therapist, the next step was making a slight pivot, then slowly lowering to the mat.

Walking is normally a fairly straightforward activity. The need to walk is recognized, the brain sends the message to the body, and then the feet and legs move. These messages from the brain happen in a split second. Walking is accomplished without the need of conscious thought. After a stroke or other brain injury that may no longer be the case. This cognitive element of retraining someone to walk is a major element that a therapist will address. When the message from the brain does not automatically occur, a person may be required to learn to send out the messages consciously. This requires a person to concentrate on movement with focus on each step in the sequence to accomplish the specific task at hand. This is an extremely strenuous process. It was important to concentrate not only on movement, but the sequence of the task as well.

In the beginning, it was impossible to complete the process of standing and getting seated on the therapy mat independently. The therapist was careful to monitor, cue, and provide physical assistance when needed through each step from standing to sitting on the mat, then back into the chair when our session was over. When she was satisfied that it was safe to begin the session, she gave careful instructions for each activity. One of the first problems to address was sitting independently. Being able to sit in an upright centered position is important for many reasons. On a personal level, being unable to sit straight was something that was extremely unpleasant. I'd always had good posture, and it was very demoralizing to be unable to maintain that aspect of myself. To begin the slow process of retraining sitting, the therapist first sat next to me using gentle pressure to hold me up. Gradually, she began placing my left hand on the mat for support. Eventually, she was able to take very brief moments of removing her assistance. After numerous successful trials, she became comfortable with allowing me a few seconds of independence, while continuing to remain close enough to prevent any potential fall that might result in an injury. In each session we worked from one exercise to another in a systematic manner targeting both upper and lower body activities. Many of the exercises were familiar from previous aerobics experiences. Unlike the days of step aerobics classes the most minor movement was incredibly difficult, if not impossible.

Every day, each therapist adjusted the number, types or intensity of the exercises according to progress and tolerance. Very slowly, the exercises progressed from getting out of the wheelchair to sit on the mat and eventually to getting out of the wheelchair in order to stand. At first this was possible only through the assistance of the physical therapist, but eventually it was possible to stand independently for short periods of time. That point began the slow process of taking a step, then eventually two steps and so on until walking with an aide was possible. The first steps were very awkward and unsteady. To assist me, the therapist provided a four footed cane to help me walk around. It was only with supervision and minor assistance at first, then gradually progressing to being on my own. That did not mean being independent. It meant being followed and watched constantly. Although understandable, it was nonetheless difficult to accept the loss of freedom, within the more or less controlled environment of the hospital.

My constant curiosity about my progress must have made every therapist crazy, but they were very understanding. Physical restoration, particularly in my left foot and leg, began rather quickly. The physical therapist commented that it was a good example of the plasticity of a "young" nervous system. At the age of forty-one, I was considered a "young stroke."

Eventually it was possible for me to walk with the cane, and we were able to work on exercises in the courtyard off to the side of the gym. This outdoor courtyard had been designed to improve mobility on a variety of surfaces. Good weather often permitted outside activities to work on walking as well as balance and stamina. If the weather did not permit working outside we continued the usual activities inside. No matter where the sessions were conducted, they included exercises designed to improve every area of my physical ability.

In addition to the usual OT and PT sessions, the two therapists developed a program of aquatic therapy as well. The wheelchair continued to be necessary, but I was eventually allowed to wheel myself to and from therapies. Exercises in the aquatic setting were free from wheelchair confinement. Aquatic therapy has many advantages. Water provides a natural resistance to movement as well as buoyancy that takes pressure away from joints. The rehabilitation exercises included using the existing water resistance, as well as adding resistance through the use of devices specifically designed for the purpose of increasing resistance to movement in water. Jerry was given the task of obtaining one of my swimsuits from home. Two piece suits were clearly out of the question. He knew my two favorite one piece suits but wasn't sure which one I would prefer for therapy. He brought both suits and it was quickly obvious that only one would be practical. One suit was a standard two arm opening style the other was halter styled. Neither would be easy for me, but the standard style was the least problematic.

Proof of a lack of connection between physical and cognitive abilities was manifested in areas of memory and attention to detail (common problems created by right hemisphere damage). Although I had a pair of "reef walkers" that were required in the pool for safety reasons, I did not always remember to wear them. Problems with attention to detail included putting my swimsuit on backwards, or being late to the session. Physical exercises continued ranging from simple to strenuous. There was also therapy to improve proprioception. Proprioception is the awareness of posture, movement, and equilibrium changes. This includes knowing weight, position, and resistance of objects in relation to the body. This allows us to walk on a variety of surfaces safely. A machine designed for the purpose of improving these skills called the "Balance Master" became an essential part of the daily routine in my physical therapy. The Balance Master is a machine with a standing platform that can simulate motion and a person must adjust their balance to the movement using an eye level screen for visual feedback. For stamina, there were sessions on a stationary bicycle.

Although it felt like forever, it became possible to walk independently at about the fourth week after rehabilitation admission. Even so, it was not possible to walk alone anywhere in the rehabilitation hospital. There continued to be constant observation and my having an escort to each therapy. It seemed to me that I was not expected to be responsible yet for getting to therapy sessions. It also appeared to me that there was an overabundant interest in my behavior, as well as some degree of concern about my ability, or perhaps willingness to reach therapy sessions independently.

A perfect example of the results of a right hemisphere stroke on higher cognitive functions occurred one evening after therapies were over. I was sitting in my room thinking about my day. Then, for some unknowable reason, I suddenly became fixated on the idea that I needed to go down to the second floor to my former office. Never stopping to consider the fact that it would not be possible to get into the office, I set off on my quest anyway. Somehow it was possible to make my way to the office unhindered. After arriving at the office door I knew that it was a mistake since I had no key to get inside. Even so, it was a few minutes before my brain registered defeat and I returned to my room. Unfortunately, but not unexpectedly, this behavior only served to put me on the "watchful eye" program. A magnet picturing a large eye and the words "watchful eye" was placed on the outside doorframe of my room. This designated me as high risk for engaging in unsafe behavior. Additionally, in order to ensure that I did not injure myself through unsafe activities or if I attempted to leave the room again, someone came every hour to look in and ask me if I was all right, or maybe see if I was actually there. I knew from my work as a therapist that this was a process developed for patient safety.

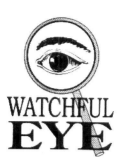

WATCHFUL EYE

One disturbing incident, unlike the fixation and poor judgment of my leaving the room, occurred one evening after having dinner with Jerry. We had said our goodbyes and good nights and he left. On that particular evening his departure caused more sadness than usual. I went to the window to see if I could catch sight of him leaving the building. I was able to see him as he walked to his car, but seeing him leave made me experience a serious episode of emotional lability (loss of emotional control). I was overcome with a rush of unhappiness that had never occurred before, for any reason. I began to cry uncontrollably. In addition, I began to think about calling him just to hear his voice, perhaps for comfort. Unfortunately, I could not consider the time lapse between his departure from the hospital and arrival at home. So, without stopping to think it through, I called our house. When the machine picked up it made me realize my mistake and, at the same time, made me even more distressed. I left him a long tearful rambling message that caused him some degree of stress.

Although it had become obvious after one or two weeks that my strength had improved, I continued to feel drained by all my activities. It did not help that I was extremely frustrated by the restrictions on my mobility and activities. I felt that I had lost my privacy and freedom as well. Although the situation was frustrating, I made an effort to accept the need for these precautions.

Like many stroke patients, my speech therapy session had been scheduled prior to lunch. Unlike some stroke patients, I was not affected by a disturbance in my ability to swallow. That meant that there was no need for a therapist to supervise or assist me with eating. This was very good because it meant that my meals could be eaten in my room. Another good thing was that patients chose meals from a menu. It was great to learn that the food was actually quite good. There was no mushy stuff or green Jell-O every day. The best thing was that Jerry could spend time with me during dinner. He even brought nonalcoholic wine to accompany my food.

The term most often used in reference to speech and language pathology (SLP) is simply "speech therapy." Communication is not limited to the act of speaking. As in other therapies addressing cognitive function, many of the speech therapy activities were on a rudimentary skill level. It was painful to recognize activities from my previous work as a therapist. In addition, it was more painful to be unable to correctly perform many of those simple, as well as familiar, tasks. Simple math problems or elementary level reading activities were too difficult for me. It was particularly disturbing to realize that in spite of the fact that I had taught memory skills for nearly five years, I could not put those skills to use during my own therapy exercises. I became distressed and frustrated about losing my previous level of ability. Additionally, it was embarrassing to recognize mistakes involving various therapy tasks. I knew that a loss of brain function made me unable to initially walk or use my left arm along with a loss of cognitive ability.

These realizations were extremely distressing. At the same time, I knew that my body would recover more quickly and far better than my intellect. In a speech therapy group the therapist used a variety of exercises designed to promote restoration of facial muscle function. These exercises coupled with those in other therapies promoted positive effects to develop over a relatively short span of time. Fortunately, I was not effected with communication problems such as aphasia. Having a right hemisphere stroke did not have an effect on either my receptive or expressive language. My problems were concerned instead with the ability to recognize nonverbal cues from other people during conversation, leading to a tendency to talk incessantly, a condition known as verboseness. In addition, a problem called tangential thinking made it difficult for me to connect subjects accurately without digressing onto unrelated topics.

Two biofeedback therapists were assigned to my team and each worked on different specific areas of need. Each of them used a computerized system designed for measurement of my muscle movements to be translated into a visual image on a computer screen. This was accomplished by connecting electrodes to targeted muscles in each session. These electrodes were used in the same manner that an EKG is performed. As my muscles moved, my impulses were relayed to a computer and converted into visual images on the computer monitor. Lifting, bending, or other movements in my limbs or face became a picture of a line on a graph with horizontal lines depicting levels of muscle movement and a line that spiked and dipped as movements were made. The more movement I made, the higher the line jumped. The line would be flat along the bottom of the screen when no movement was made.

The first therapy session began with the therapist setting our goal as working to make movements that would create a smile. As she pointed to a line on the screen, she said, "This is how the graph looks when you are sitting still." Pointing to another line she said, "This is where you want the line to be." When compared to this "baseline" measure, the goal appeared to be very high. Each successive session with either therapist began in a similar fashion by working on various muscle groups and comparing a baseline of activity to a goal. In both cases it was obvious that reaching the targeted goal would require not only a lengthy period of time, but a great deal of work as well. Return of function begins in the large muscle groups and slowly progresses to the small muscle groups. Therefore, therapy began by concentrating on small movements involving gross motor (large muscle) activities such as lifting my left arm from the shoulder or lifting my leg. When we were able to progress to smaller muscles, I was asked to move the corners of my mouth or to move my hand or fingers up and down until the graph changed. It felt as if a one hundred-pound weight was attached to each finger by invisible threads so that lifting my hand was transformed into lifting five hundred pounds. Lifting each finger only isolated one of the hundred pound weights.

Similarly, the same type of invisible weight pulled the left side of my face downward from hairline to chin. In the beginning there was no movement at all on the graphs in either biofeedback therapy session. It seemed that the measurement line would remain flat on the bottom of the screen forever.

Finally, being able to make movement and causing the line to spike up into the first level of measurement seemed like an enormous accomplishment. That accomplishment was also reinforcement for continuing to work for higher goals. During these sessions my concentration became focused on the computer screen. Since my ability to concentrate had been reduced by the stroke, this therapy method benefited me in concentration, as well as muscle movement. Like all therapies, every movement took so much effort that I was exhausted at the end of each session. An unpleasant part of the biofeedback therapy was removing the electrodes and the sticky conduction fluid.

I was assured at the end of each session that my progress was good. I knew that progress was being made because changes in the biofeedback graphs were obvious. Yet, looking in the mirror, there seemed to be little evidence that my facial or limb muscles were improving. Lopsidedness remained even into the fourth week of my rehabilitation therapy. Leg movement and support had significantly improved by about the fourth week. Still, my arm movement had not returned; it remained limp and unresponsive. Smiling was beginning to show change but seemed so much less than normal. There also seemed to be no improvement in automatic responses in my physical or cognitive behaviors. My spontaneity of expression and verbal responses along with voice quality remained seriously impaired. These facts validated concerns about the serious level of damage to the deep areas of my brain responsible for automatic (involuntary) functions.

In addition to OT, PT, SLP, and biofeedback, it was decided that cognitive rehabilitation would be appropriate. The task of choosing a therapist for cognitive rehabilitation therapy was particularly difficult. Each therapist was a direct colleague of mine and the dual relationship issue was too difficult to overcome. Therefore, it was decided that the best choice would be to find an outside source. The therapist chosen to provide my cognitive rehabilitation therapy was an independent provider who was not associated with Genesis.

This therapist and I met in my hospital room the Friday prior to our first session in order to become aquatinted and establish rapport. Although she was no older than I, she had a number of years of experience with a broad range of people who had various types of brain injuries. We were required to work within the confines of my hospital room until the time of my discharge. Although this presented a variety of challenges, we were able to make the best of things.

On May 1st, Jerry and I would celebrate the tenth year of our relationship. We had always celebrated our anniversary and we decided that our tenth should not go unmarked. I was walking by then, but had not been out of or away from the hospital for any reason other than therapy. We asked permission to be allowed an outing together to celebrate our anniversary by going out to dinner. The pros and cons of such an idea had to be weighed carefully. Still, Jerry had proven himself as a responsible caregiver and the therapists and physician agreed that it would be very therapeutic. After many discussions and evaluations we were given permission for an outing. Jerry made a reservation at an upscale restaurant and brought me clothes and accessories that I requested. While we were able to enjoy a good dinner and had a nice time, it was not at all like a normal celebration. We had a curfew along with many limitations on activities. It was impossible for either of us to be completely relaxed. Still, the evening went well. The restaurant was one we had been to before, but not for a while. It was well known for its seafood selections, so we were able to enjoy our favorites. Jerry had the sea bass and I had the snapper. We did not get any wine with dinner. I did have to return to the hospital, after all, and Jerry had to drive. After dinner, Jerry drove me back to Genesis. As I approached the nurse's station to let them know that I had returned, the nurse on duty, a different one from when I left earlier, seemed shocked to learn that I was a patient.

After six weeks of therapy, discharge became imminent. Discharge would not mean the end of therapy. The physical problems of paralysis, balance, and strength loss had resolved to a functional level but cognition remained significantly impaired. My strength, although functional, was not at a pre-stroke level but it was good enough that I no longer required the intensive activity of the hospital.

In preparation for discharge, each therapist made evaluations to assess my progress toward the goals set in the rehabilitation plan. The physical therapist evaluated my ability to walk on a variety of surfaces, stand on one foot, run a short distance, and use stairs safely. She also tested stamina and balance skills. The occupational therapist tested various degrees of arm and hand strength and dexterity as well as cognitive skills. In order to test cognition in areas of independent living skills, a cooking evaluation was required. Cooking requires planning and follow through, logic, judgment, and many other cognitive skills. Simple meal preparation is a common method not only for assessment of these skills, but is a matter of practicality for someone being discharged from a hospital setting to an independent situation. Luckily, the assessment would focus on a moderate level cooking activity. Working with the occupational therapist, she and I planned a full dinner menu which included three courses. I chose a spaghetti dinner and so we planned a meal that included salad, spaghetti, and chocolate mousse for dessert. It was well known that I enjoyed cooking. Knowing that the cooking activity would be a close look at many cognitive skills that were compromised by my stroke, however, was somewhat troublesome. Success or failure would have an impact on my discharge plans and recommendations from the therapist and made me worry about my ability to perform well. When the time came for the cooking evaluation, the OT, PT, and I had completed the shopping for each part of the meal. Jerry brought my KitchenAid hand mixer and a Paul Prudhomme cookbook to the hospital so that it would be easy to make the chocolate mousse.

As we entered the kitchen, I realized that I had not cooked anything in quite some time so it would be different in more ways than simply being in a kitchen that was unfamiliar to me. The OT looked at the clock and said, "Well, looks like you're good to go." I made a quick survey of the kitchen, then began to lay out the ingredients for the spaghetti.

Stepping back, I checked the list from a recipe that we had chosen. Feeling satisfied that everything was correct, I picked up the onion and inspected it. The OT asked me if I thought it was good. I told her that it was and I began removing the outer layers. I tossed the onion skins into the trash can and set the onion experimentally on the counter. The OT said, "I know what you're thinking." I smiled and said, "Sure you do, you know I'm thinking about chopping this onion." She replied, "Yes, and you probably want a cutting board." I told her that she was right, and that I did need a cutting board. Then she said, "You don't want just any cutting board, you need a special one." She walked to a cabinet, reached into it and took out a cutting board with a single spike jutting out of it. She placed the board on the counter and waited to see if I would figure out how to use it. My left arm and hand were still a bit weak so I held the onion with both hands and allowed her to guide me to get the onion onto the spike to begin cutting. I went to the knife block that was near the end of the counter and chose a knife that I felt would work well for my purpose. I cut the onion using the technique that I had learned many years before from one source or another. By making horizontal and vertical slices fully across the onion, into a checkerboard fashion, then slicing downward, I created a medium dice. After that, we moved on to the actual cooking. While the sauce simmered, I went to work on the mousse. By then both the OT and PT were observing me. Although it made me a little nervous, I knew it was necessary. The PT picked up the Prudhomme cookbook and read the inscription inside. She remarked, "Looks like you've had this book a while." I told her that, "Yes, it's been around for a while and I've made a few things from it and I have never been disappointed with any of the recipes." I had made the mousse many times so luckily, there were no problems. When everything was over, I felt a sense of accomplishment that I hoped was warranted. It turned out, the meal was deemed a success by both the OT and PT.

Subsequently, plans were made for discharge from Genesis tentatively on May 12, 1995. Based on evaluations that had been performed by the therapists, it was recommended that I continue therapy at the hospital's main outpatient center on a three days a week schedule. It was determined that my physical recovery, although excellent, would benefit from further physical therapy and that cognitive skills should be addressed through occupational therapy, as well as speech and language pathology and cognitive rehabilitation therapies.

Just as the therapists had completed evaluations of physical and cognitive functions, administrators tackled the logistical problems of providing a continuation of the recommended therapies. A major consideration was transportation to not only the outpatient center, but to the office of the independent cognitive rehabilitation therapist as well. To further complicate things, a weekly trip to a lab for blood work, for continued monitoring of the anticoagulant level, was needed. In the end, all the plans seemed to be in order and we could look forward to continuation of therapy at the outpatient center and at the office of the cognitive rehabilitation therapist. I knew that I was very far from being done with therapy and, although that was disheartening, it was not realistic to think about it being over.

Chapter 4—Outpatient Therapy

My discharge day at Genesis had been busy and in many ways confusing. Since nurses and doctors met mostly with Jerry for my paperwork, my involvement had been minimal. My main concern had been packing things up to go home. After six weeks, there was a substantial accumulation of clothing and toiletry items to be packed. It was difficult to keep track of what was packed and what was waiting for packing. Eventually it seemed that every item was packaged in one way or another for travel. After paperwork and recommendations had been completed, the nurses, therapists, and doctors came to wish me good luck and hopes for better days ahead. We were given a three ring binder full of exercises and activities intended to continue therapeutic activities after discharge. I knew about this binder because, as a previous team member, we had developed what we hoped would be a tool for patients to use after discharge for continuation of some level of rehabilitation at home.

Finally, we began our departure taking as much in each hand as we could manage. Jerry took the bulk of it due to the continued weakness on my left side. We made it out of the building and to the car without great difficulty. When we began packing the car we both realized that we had left a few things in the room. Jerry quickly made a return trip to the room to retrieve the missing items. When everything was finally loaded, we left for home. It was so good to be out in the world again and I was happy to finally be returning to our home.

Since there would be a full week break between discharge from the hospital and the start of outpatient therapy, Jerry made arrangements for leave time to stay home with me during that period. While we were not totally convinced that the recommendations of the therapists for constant supervision were completely necessary, we remained concerned about continued problems of logic, judgment, problem solving, and short-term memory. With that in mind, we decided that it would be better for Jerry to stay home rather than me being at home alone so soon after discharge. In addition, we felt that it would be best for me to refrain from driving. Although it was an unpleasant thought, it was acceptable. It would be inconvenient for us and stressful for Jerry, but we decided that it would be best to wait for further improvements from therapy as well as evaluations from therapists.

Surprisingly, adjusting to the lack of structured activity proved to be more difficult than we could have anticipated. The stroke had stripped away my enthusiasm, self- directed behavior, as well as energy and ambition. Although I was happy to finally be at home, it was not the same as an illness causing me to stay at home away from work. Prior to the stroke it would have been easy to find numerous projects to complete with so much free time. By the end of that week, returning to therapy began to look more attractive than it had at the time of hospital discharge. Finally, it was time to prepare for continuation of therapy at the outpatient center. On Monday, a transportation van from Genesis arrived promptly at 9:15 a.m. in order to assure arrival at the center on schedule for the first therapy session at 10:00 a.m.

The van ride seemed bumpy, and was new and strange to me. Surprisingly, there were only one or two other patients making the trip with me. After arriving at the outpatient center, the first thing to do was meet the therapists, some I had never met before. The positive aspects of working with the outpatient therapists was that they were less familiar to me and me to them. Fortunately, they were as professional as those with whom I had previously worked as an inpatient. They were adept at their jobs and tried their best to make me feel comfortable in the new situation. Many therapy activities continued to be at a very low level of difficulty for the average person. The level of recovery of cognitive functions was a constant concern. Continued goals for physical therapy were to improve strength, stamina, coordination, and balance. Occupational and speech therapies included a continuation of physical activities in addition to goals for improvement of particular cognitive skills such as problem solving, logic, organization, and memory skills. All therapies were a steady progression of difficult physical exercises and rudimentary cognitive activities. In addition to the gross motor strengthening exercises, fine motor tasks such as simple painting or woodworking were also used. While math and various other cognitive work seemed simplistic, they proved to be difficult nonetheless. While efforts were made to maintain the planned transportation to and from a lab once each week for blood-work, and transport to the off-site office of the cognitive rehabilitation therapist, things did not always run smoothly, but no appointments or treatment sessions were missed.

As time passed, my physical abilities continued to improve to a more functional level. In spite of the strong physical activities provided by the therapists, I missed being able to attend step-aerobics classes. Eventually, I approached the physical therapist with the idea of allowing me to attend a class only once a week. After discussing the issue with my physiatrist, the therapist agreed that I would be allowed to attend the low impact class once a week. Naturally, there was a catch. Assuming that blood pressure problems were a factor in my stroke, she would require that my blood pressure be monitored before and after the class to insure that I could tolerate the activity level. This puzzled me because I knew that my blood pressure was not a factor in my stroke, according to my neurologist.

My blood pressure had always been low. I was pronounced with a "runners pulse" by at least two of my previous physicians. It was unpleasant to accept the terms for my participation in an aerobics class. It seemed that it was more important to take advantage of the opportunity in spite of the restrictions. The blood pressure issue would prove to be the least unpleasant aspect of the aerobics class. It was difficult to approach the first class without a degree of apprehension. Although I felt ready to participate, I was also intimidated. Still, I attended the class. Unfortunately, there were cognitive issues related to my stroke that I had not considered. The physical aspect of the class was of little difficulty. Cognitive changes made the activity not only more difficult, but unpleasant as well. The music that had previously been so enjoyable was suddenly reduced to nothing more than noise. Getting coordinated with the beat or tempo was impossible. Attempting to compensate for remaining problems with left side neglect only served to create problems in maintaining any sense of spatial relations. Wildly bouncing around from spot to spot made for more than one near crash into another class participant. In addition, my stroke made my perception of the instructor's voice sound grating.

The combination of attending to music, the instructor, and the floor space was too much to contend with. The once pleasant class experience was a total disaster that left me feeling demoralized and unhappy. Waiting in line with the elderly cardiac patients for a blood pressure check topped off the experience in a negative way. The combination of these elements gave me little impetus to continue, and after a few classes, I gave up the effort. This would not have happened prior to the stroke. I had always been more determined to succeed rather than give up. My first exposure to group aerobic activity had been when I was much younger, when Jazzercise became popular, it had seemed unlikely that it would be possible to participate, but rather than give up I made it a habit.

As July approached it was decided by my therapy team that it would be beneficial to have some in-depth neuropsychological information to help them direct my therapy to the most necessary areas. I had suspected that it would eventually be necessary to undergo a full neuropsychological evaluation for the purpose of assessing my progress and to determine further therapy needs, as well as to set discharge goals. The close nature of my relationships with the neuropsychologists at Genesis, who would normally conduct the neuropsychological testing, once again made it necessary to obtain services elsewhere. One of the neuropsychologists at Genesis suggested some other places and gave us contact information to make arrangements. We contacted a neuropsychologist to set up an appointment for administering the evaluation. Having the neuropsychological evaluation completed by someone unfamiliar was a positive thing. Making a drive to another town, however, was not entirely positive. Jerry and I discussed the issue several times before making our final plans to travel for the evaluation. The order for my testing stated that the purpose of the testing would be to assist the interdisciplinary rehabilitation team in tailoring therapy to address my goal of returning to work.

Luckily, we had been given very specific directions to our destination. Even so, the maze of halls, offices and the volume of people were more than enough for anyone to manage. We were concerned that it would be impossible to find our way out of the building, much less back to the car, when it came time to leave. In spite of the confusion, we managed to locate the check-in area and get all the necessary paperwork completed without incident. When the paperwork was completed, I was given a simple ID card specifying basic personal information and my purpose at the hospital. After a brief wait, a person arrived and escorted us to the testing area. Once we arrived at the testing room we met with the neuropsychologist to go over the process with us. I was nervous because I knew that my intellectual performance would be evaluated.

The next day we returned to the hospital and the neuropsychologist explained what the testing revealed. As would generally be expected with right hemisphere damage, I learned that my cognitive difficulties continued. I had problems such as minimal affective reactions (facial expressions) and poor perceptual-organizational and constructional abilities (seeing the whole from the parts). Fortunately, strengths were in the areas of language. Overall, lost skills had improved in relation to the initial screening completed immediately after the stroke, but continued to be below my expected pre-stroke ability levels. The neuropsychologist gave recommendations to the outpatient therapists that included structured, supervised work-related activity in preparation for discharge from therapy and returning to work. The neuropsychologist emphasized that he was unable to confidently predict that I would be successful when I returned to work. I listened to the results of the tests with mixed feelings. It was disheartening to hear that my skills were lowered in the performance areas of the test. Although it was difficult to face, I knew that the changes were the result of damage to the right hemisphere of my brain. It was encouraging to learn that my language functions continued to be high. Language has always been one of my strongest abilities.

In August, the therapists began to discuss discharge from outpatient therapy. The cognitive rehabilitation therapist and I talked about my goal of returning to work and the recommendations of the neuropsychologist. She made a plan to involve me in some work-related activities in preparation for going back to work. In addition, she talked to me about returning to driving. We also discussed the inevitability of a driving evaluation by a Genesis therapist trained for that purpose. After one or two work-related cognitive therapy sessions it appeared that I still had a small degree of competence in therapy delivery. Still, the activity itself presented tremendous strain on not only cognition, but my physical state as well. It was so exhausting that my stamina gave out after only 30 minutes. I told the therapist that the only experience with similar physically draining activities was my teaching internship in college.

After she had made several assessments of the job-related activities, she suggested that it might be wise to think about some preparation for a driving evaluation. That, apparently, was not a goal of the therapists at the outpatient center. They were not yet enthusiastic about the idea of my driving, or going back to work.

Driving seemed especially difficult to consider. In light of the fact that I had a right hemisphere stroke, my own concerns made me reluctant to get back to driving. Seeing the reluctance of the therapists to my driving made it more difficult for me to think about driving as well. In a large city where mass transit services are available, not driving would be a lesser problem. Where public transportation is limited driving is a necessity. The cognitive rehabilitation therapist eventually convinced me that it would be wise to at least assess my memory of the sequence of events to start a car. To that end, she planned a few therapy sessions to explore those initial elements of driving. First she required a review of the driving manual and a test on road rules and signs.

When she felt that I was ready to work toward our goal, we went to the parking lot and got into her car. In the first session, the only thing she wanted to find out was whether I could correctly complete the initial sequence to prepare for driving (setting mirrors, seatbelt, etc.). For a minute, I was very disoriented. I did not think about the fact that the last time I was in a car to drive had been the Friday before my stroke. Getting into this strange car was very unusual. I spent a good minute just looking at the interior. I glanced down on the left and felt a shock when I did not see a clutch. She started to laugh and I looked at her and said, "Oh yes, I'm looking for my clutch." She said, "You won't find one in this car." I had to laugh also, and said, "Maybe because this isn't my car?" "Very good", she said.

When she was satisfied after two test sessions that I could do the basic things, she gave me the keys and had me drive around the parking lot and then re-park the car. This created a concern at the outpatient center. This did not surprise me. In my experience, occasional differences of opinion were not uncommon among professionals. A therapist told me that driving instruction and assessments were the sole property of one particular therapy (not cognitive rehabilitation therapy) and should not be dealt with by anyone outside that discipline. The cognitive rehabilitation therapist had not provided a driving evaluation, only a cursory review of the most basic elements of driving.

I was glad that I had been given the opportunity to be exposed to driving prior to taking the official driving evaluation with the OT. I was better prepared and had a little more confidence. I was scared, but I knew I would have to drive before I could return to work. Thankfully, I passed the exam with only minor suggestions from the examiner. One of her recommendations was to drive faster (more to the speed limit). She said I was "driving like a little old lady." This was very strange since I generally had no difficulty with speed. I tended to have a lead foot. I think I inherited it from my father, who loved cars and loved to drive. I had fond memories of driving the latest model Nissan Z cars when I worked one summer for the Nissan dealership in Milton, FL. Driving slowly was quite new for me.

Although I passed the sessions and felt that I would not kill anyone or myself due to my impairments, driving did not seem as natural as it had before my stroke. The pleasure of driving was taken away by my stroke. In spite of that, it was good to know that I would be able to drive to work, if and when the time came. Although it was encouraging to know that driving was not impossible, it did not cause me to get excited and impatient to begin driving right away. At that time I remained skeptical of my competence. I did not feel as comfortable in the car or with the feel of speed, unlike my days before my stroke when speed was not only comfortable but preferable. I was convinced that I would eventually return to work. It did not seem to me that anyone would decide that I could not go back.

Because therapy was not officially over, I had to continue therapy at the outpatient center as well as the independent cognitive rehabilitation therapist's office. Since I was cleared to drive, I was no longer required to ride in the van. I had to get to those places on my own. It did not worry me that this was the case. I felt that if I started driving and did it routinely, it would become more natural and less stressful. My only concern was figuring out the easiest route to and from each place. Fortunately, Jerry was able to help me drive the easiest route a couple of times. Still, every day I had to work to remember exactly what route I had to take. Although I would be in the right place, sometimes the streets and surroundings looked unfamiliar and it made me worry.

It was not always easy to feel comfortable during any particular trip. As it turned out, I was generally on time for therapies. Although I had a cell phone, it was only for emergency situations. I would not ever use it while driving. It was a rule that I never broke. Luckily, no emergencies occurred while making trips to and from therapies. The toll on my stamina was significant and made it necessary to rest in the therapist's office before heading out to my next destination. This was especially true after a work simulation with the cognitive rehabilitation therapist. She often made me take a break and drink water before she would allow me to leave her office. Although this was an effective solution to the problem, it did not bolster my confidence. It did, however, give an indication of one more problem to be dealt with resulting from my stroke. It was not easy to have a positive attitude about all of these things. What had once been so easy was now terribly difficult.

While having work simulations to prepare for returning to my job was a good thing, it was also strange. During teaching internships students are observed and graded on their work. In therapy it was not only being scrutinized, but also tested. At first it was particularly difficult to take on the therapist position, while being a patient at the same time. The therapist was very considerate of this unusual situation and did not make constant suggestions or interrupt a session with critical feedback. Still, it was hard to focus on giving therapy while being observed directly. It was only after a session that she would go over her notes with me regarding her observations. She first noted the drain on my energy during our earliest work simulation session. She had communicated this observation to the other therapists at the outpatient center so that they would be able to make necessary accommodations. They were good at listening to her suggestions. As the outpatient period was coming to an end, it was helpful to have everyone coordinating efforts toward my goal of returning to work.

Chapter 5—Hi Ho, Hi Ho!

The route to my profession as a cognitive rehabilitation therapist was a circuitous one that marginally related to my degree in elementary education. My mother has always had a strong commitment to ensuring that my sisters and I would be able to go to college. Due to her efforts, I was able to begin my educational journey after high school beginning with Pensacola Junior College (currently Pensacola State College). I knew that I would pursue a degree in elementary education, from the beginning of my college experiences, when I took an Introduction to Education course.

By a chance invitation from a friend, I went to a student-recruiting visit at the University of South Florida (USF) in the spring of 1974, just prior to completion of coursework for an Associate of Arts degree at Pensacola Junior College. While I was wandering around through some exhibits from the various programs, I stopped at the display for the College of Education. A faculty member came over and asked me if I was planning to attend the university and if I would be attending the College of Education. Although I had not made a firm decision in either case, I impulsively (reflexively) said, "Yes" to both questions. That particular impulsive response turned out to be one of the most important positive results of my instinctual reactions.

The teacher told me some of the good aspects of attending USF, and then he asked me if I had any problems with which he might be able to help. I told him that I would want to work while I was attending the university. He thought for a moment, then told me that he knew of a program called "impact aides" that would add teacher aides to lower level elementary classes. The program was scheduled to begin in local elementary schools in the fall of that year. He asked me if I was interested in a job as an aide. I told him that I was, and he gave me a job application to take with me. He then asked me if I wanted to live on campus or if I would consider living off campus. He told me he knew some students who needed a housemate. I decided that I would take a chance on that, and he gave me their names and phone numbers. I went away with the knowledge that I would get a degree in elementary education at USF, and get some experience with elementary school students at the same time. This was not a feeling, it was a confirmation. It seemed clear to me that I was supposed to attend USF and become a teacher. When I think back about that time I say, "It's too bad there was no lottery back then." It was the best luck I could have had.

After I returned home, I made the appropriate contacts for employment and living arrangements. To my surprise, I was quickly hired as a teacher's aide at an elementary school that happened to be close to the University. I was also accepted as a housemate with three female students who had a house in Temple Terrace, a quiet section of town also close to the University. My job at the elementary school required that I be in Tampa in August. University courses, however, would not begin until September. True to my independent nature, when it was time to leave home, I had no difficulty. I left with only the verbal directions that my father gave me. Nevertheless, his directions were as accurate as any map. Although he may have had some reservations about my leaving for school, he was quite helpful in preparing me for the trip. I did not have a car at that time, so prior to preparing to leave, he went about finding a car for me. He found a very interesting car somewhere in Pensacola. He told me that he had found a car that he thought I might like and that he would bring it home as soon as he could. He cautioned that I would have the responsibility of making the payments for it.

When he finally brought the car home, it was a surprise. It was not a make or model that was familiar. It was very interesting because it was a British car called Austin America. As soon as I sat in the seat it was clear that it was my car. For one thing, it was small; the other features of interest were its vertical speedometer and multi-purpose steering column. The steering column included, not only the customary turn signals and windshield wipers, but the headlight controls and the horn as well. It was also a standard transmission. The paint was "British racing green," according to the paperwork. Not only was it perfect for me to drive, it got very good gas mileage. Interstate 10 (I-10) had not been completed at that time so the early part of my journey would be on Hwy 90. Although I took several different highways, it was a surprisingly easy drive into Tampa. I had the directions to the house in Temple Terrace, and I drove directly to the house to meet my new housemates. When I arrived there I must have been very nervous. When I parked in the slightly slanted driveway to the house, I forgot to put on the emergency brake. As I was talking to one of the students at the door, my car began rolling into the street. I ran to catch it, but even if I had been large enough or strong enough, it would have been difficult at best to stop it. Fortunately, due to a lack of air conditioning, the window was open so I managed to turn the steering wheel so that the car would be close to the curb and parallel to the house. Thankfully, it stopped on its own with the leveling out of the street. It was a strange introduction to my new living arrangements. The other students probably laughed about it later, but I don't know for sure. Nevertheless, I got settled into my room and began to aquatint myself with the other girls.

The next week it was necessary for me to drive into downtown Tampa for fingerprinting prior to working at the elementary school. I wondered what my overly protective parents would say if they knew that I would be driving there. Up to that point in my life, my driving experience was somewhat limited. When I set out to drive to Tampa, it was clear that my parents would be extremely worried the entire time until I called them to say that I had arrived safely. As it turned out, my trip was quite uneventful. Likewise, when I went to the courthouse in downtown Tampa things went just as smoothly. In spite of the rocky start at the house, everything worked out beautifully. I earned my Bachelor of Arts degree and enjoyed excellent experience in an elementary school at the same time. Not only did it solidify my decision to become a teacher, it was my most useful college experience.

At the time of my graduation, teaching positions were limited all over Florida. Thinking that it would be just as easy to wait for a position in my hometown of Milton as it would be in Tampa, I chose to return to Milton. From 1976 to 1979 while looking for a teaching position, I worked at a variety of jobs. I was also able to take a temporary job as a kindergarten teacher. After a year without success in finding a permanent teaching position, I returned to school at the University of West Florida (UWF) to earn certification in an area of special education with the hope that I could improve my chances of finding a teaching position. Along the way I worked as a tutor through the University, a waitress at a local country club, and in a small, but rowdy, Pensacola bar. One summer I had a sporadic job of driving cars for the Nissan dealership in Milton where my father worked as a salesman. When it was necessary to exchange one car for another in some other town, I might be called to make the drive. The work was off and on but it was a great deal of fun to drive a variety of new cars from one place to another. The furthest trips were only to places like Dothan, Alabama or Panama City, Florida. I also worked for a short time in a daycare center, and as a sales clerk in a small clothing store in downtown Pensacola.

Finally, in 1979, I got a break with another turn of events. The Santa Rosa Association for Retarded Citizens (ARC) needed a teacher in their sheltered workshop. Someone from the ARC made a visit to the school board office to review applications of prospective teachers. He asked to see as many applications as possible. After reaching the end of the files he was given, he asked if there were any other files. He was directed to a group of files that he was told were the applications of people considered unsuitable for their schools. Nevertheless, he looked at those files also. That is where he found my application.

At that time, the clothing shop where I worked as a sales clerk abruptly closed. About a week later, on a Friday afternoon, I was called regarding the teaching position at the ARC. I was asked to come in for an interview the following week. I was hired for the job and began very soon afterward. At the time, the position was only ten hours a week. That was not a problem because I was told it would change over time. At first, I was wary about the position at the ARC. Although I had the necessary education and training, I did not have any practical experience in the area of developmental disabilities. That situation did not last long. I grew into the job and remained in the position until 1989. By that time, the position had grown to a full forty hours per week. While working at the ARC, I underwent a multitude of changes both professionally and personally. My confidence grew along with my experience. As I became more professional and mature, I was a much better employee than when I first started.

In the early 80's, another turn of events came when the Executive Director of the ARC told me that he believed that I should take on more responsibility. He suggested that I consider doing some volunteer work related to developmental disabilities. I took his suggestion and became a volunteer for Special Olympics. Later, I became a volunteer with an advocacy group for the rights of the developmentally disabled for Northwest Florida. This would lead to my meeting Jerry in his position as the State Program Administrator for the developmentally disabled in Northwest Florida. Over time we developed a good working relationship and eventually, Jerry asked me out on a date. We grew to enjoy each other's company and eventually moved into a condo in Pensacola together.

Early in 1989, Jerry and I discussed the idea of taking a different direction in our respective careers. In that spring, we were offered an opportunity to not only change our jobs, but our residence as well. The jobs we were offered would take us to the state of New Hampshire working for a brain injury rehabilitation company. The idea of such a geographical change made me think twice about such a move. I did not have any experience with very cold weather, so the thought of New Hampshire was a bit difficult to consider. Jerry, on the other hand, had lived in Boston and Minneapolis so he felt more prepared. In addition to those concerns was the fact that I was in the final stage of completing work for my MA degree in Education at the University of West Florida. Another complication was that we were renting a house in the North Hill area of Pensacola. We had convinced the owner to grant us a lease with the option to buy. That put us in an awkward position with respect to such an abrupt change in plans.

In order to complete my Master's coursework, it would be necessary for me to remain in Florida while Jerry went on to New Hampshire. At the end of the term, I would leave Pensacola and join him in New

Hampshire and work at a brain injury rehabilitation facility there. This would be my first work with brain injury rehabilitation and an introduction to the various rehabilitation therapists that work to help people with brain injuries. I knew this would mean returning to Pensacola at a later date to take my comprehensive finals, but I also knew that would not be a problem. The only negative aspect was that Jerry and I would be separated for a brief time. Still, the job opportunity was a good one, so we decided to be brave and take a chance in spite of any problems we might face as a result. At the end of the summer, I left Pensacola to join Jerry in New Hampshire for a very different job from teaching. Unfortunately, in spite of all the good people we met and worked with there, after about eight months on the job we both became dissatisfied with living in New Hampshire. We both agreed that we would return to Florida. We moved to the Jacksonville area of Florida without hesitation or reservations. Very soon after we had settled into Ponte Vedra Beach, I began working for the Duval County school system as a special education teacher. Jerry took a position in developmental disabilities with the State of Florida as a psychologist.

One Friday afternoon in the fall of 1990, when I arrived home from work, Jerry had the newspaper in his hand and he said, "I found you a job." I said, "I've got a job." He said, "You need this one. It'll be good for you." The ad described a position available for a cognitive rehabilitation therapist at Memorial Hospital in their brain injury rehabilitation program. Because he had worked in a rehabilitation center in a hospital at some previous point in his life, he always said that I needed to experience working in a hospital too. I did not know exactly what the title cognitive rehabilitation therapist meant, but it sounded interesting. Brain injury rehabilitation was familiar to me from my previous job in New Hampshire. Nevertheless, that particular therapist title was unfamiliar.

I approached the application and interview process with some excitement and a little uncertainty. Aside from one summer of volunteer work at age fifteen as a Red Cross "candy striper," I had never worked in a hospital. I had enjoyed my previous work experiences, but I was afraid that it wouldn't be enough to meet all the job requirements. In addition, the idea of working with the various other professionals that the job would naturally require intimidated me. I had some knowledge of their respective fields, but had limited exposure to them in a professional capacity from my work in New Hampshire. It made me feel that these individuals would know so much more than I did. I certainly had no experience or preparation for working alongside physicians and nurses. Yet, my experiences while working with people with developmental disabilities, as well as brain injuries, were good. It made me comfortable knowing that my training and experience were good. The uncertainty came from wondering whether it would be enough to be able do all the things that the therapist job required. There was the exciting prospect that I would learn a lot from doctors, nurses, and other therapists.

It made me extremely happy when they made the decision to hire me in November of 1990. After I began working, there was a brief period when I felt some anxiety about my ability to adapt my training to such a different population. My job in New Hampshire had been administrative rather than clinical. My previous experience in teaching had been in developmental disabilities. The hospital environment, as well as the serious medical conditions of the different patients, was very different from anything I had seen. At that time, the cognitive rehabilitation therapists worked through the Hospital's Department of Psychology under a neuropsychologist. That, at least, was something I knew about. I had met neuropsychologists during the course of my work in New Hampshire. At the hospital I would be required to work under the supervision of the neuropsychologist. I knew very quickly that I had a great deal to learn. Still, it was a very exciting time for me. It was a constant challenge to adapt my training to suit the needs of a different group of people.

In the beginning, I needed to learn the sequela of brain injury recovery and how to assess a patient's progress. In order to assess a patient's progression during the recovery process, the tool we used was the Rancho Los Amigos Rating Scale. The Rancho Scales are used to measure progress through the early stages of recovery. There were also the Glasgow Coma Scale and coma stimulation protocols for me to learn. My work would involve providing cognitive exercises as well as coma stimulation.

I learned that recovery is characterized by a progression of phases with particular behaviors in each phase. For severe head injuries (including strokes) a coma state may result. A coma may be very brief or very lengthy. While in a coma state, a person may, or may not, respond to stimulation such as lights, noises, smells, or touch. As the coma state begins to resolve, responses as well as behaviors begin to change. At first, there may only be behavior that is non-purposeful or not in response to any specific stimulation. Later, there may be a very high level of activity, but not necessarily appropriate or in accordance with the environment. By observing a patient's response to certain activities or stimulation, it is possible to determine what phase of recovery the person has reached. Many times, watching a patient progress through the various stages was fascinating.

Each patient was so different that it was a constant necessity to adapt and learn. There were some instances when a person's medical condition was so serious that they hovered on the brink of death. It was very intimidating to imagine that a person might die at any time while in my care. My instincts usually gave me a sense of how the person would progress. On occasion it seemed that instinct was only wishful thinking. Luckily, no one expired during a therapy session.

The early phases of recovery can be the most difficult for family members. During a phase of confusion, a person's behavior may be drastically different from their usual behaviors. It is difficult for family members to observe the changed behaviors without fearing the worst. It can also be difficult to accept the idea that the person is not purposely acting strangely. If a person has a temporary loss of memory for previously familiar people, it may be perceived as a deliberate act or a change of feelings.

In addition to my clinical work with the patients, it was important for me to be able to educate family members about my work to help them understand the process of recovery and the status of their family member. It was also necessary for me to learn various aspects of medical treatment from nurses and physicians. When I wasn't reading or being trained by the neuropsychologist, I was observing other therapists or asking doctors and nurses a multitude of questions. I eventually learned to work with patients to the satisfaction of my supervisor and coworkers. In addition, I reached a level of comfort about my ability as a therapist. I also learned how to communicate with the medical staff to benefit my knowledge and develop my therapy skills. Another challenge was learning how to make reports about patient progress during weekly team meetings, with all the therapists, and the physician and nurses involved in the treatment of each patient. Although it was very odd at first, I was eventually comfortable with my knowledge of my patient's status and was able to effectively communicate the necessary information to the other team members. At first the team meetings were extremely intimidating, but eventually the gregarious and open nature of the staff made the experience enjoyable. There was a professional camaraderie among us all that sometimes made the serious state of a meeting dissolve momentarily into a bit of fun and ease the tension. After a time, it was clear that the periodic playfulness of the group was in no way disrespectful toward our duties, to each other, or to our patients.

At first I found the elements of levity a bit difficult to understand. I've always been a bit too serious. Jerry often chides me about it and has frequently said, "Get over yourself." In spite of my lesser status as a new therapist, I was eventually able to earn the respect of my colleagues through my abilities and my communication skills in the many professional situations my position required. I gained a reputation for being very professional and for making accurate clinical judgements about the status of my patients at any given point in their therapy. At one point in the 90's our focus turned from a multi-disciplinary style to an interdisciplinary style. Set teams were created with each therapy represented to work together for better patient outcomes. I was asked to be a team leader for one of the brain injury teams. This was a surprise to me since I did not feel that my skills or experience were as good as some of the other therapists. Still, it was a privilege to have such support from my colleagues.

While my training and experience were the foundation of my skills, my ever accurate intuitive ability applied to my professional life as much as my personal life and was critical to my ability to make clinical judgements about any patient's progress. My gut feelings were rarely incorrect. It was imperative in my position to make accurate judgements about patient progress and to adapt therapy activities to accommodate the changing needs of patients during the course of their recovery from serious injuries to their brains. My job had a perfect balance of stimulation and challenge. It provided me with the opportunity to constantly improve and evolve into a strong, capable professional. I was happy and satisfied with my work and the work environment as well. At the end of the day there was a sense of doing something worthwhile.

Then in 1995, the stroke brought my career as a therapist to a screeching halt. After my months of therapy, I was anxious to get back to my job. At the same time, I had a number of reservations about going back to Genesis and trying to resume my job after my five-month absence and having spent time there as a patient. Additionally, I was more than a little worried about my ability to continue to work at my previous level of competency. In order to return to work, it was necessary to be evaluated by my physiatrist. After seeing him in late August, he gave me release to return to my position.

My lowered stamina continued to be a problem, so my doctor recommended a shorter workday to accommodate my need to minimize exertion. Before I could return to work, it would also be necessary to meet with my supervisor to go over the doctor's recommendations and to make arrangements for me to return to work. In accordance with the doctor's recommendation, my supervisor agreed to allow me a shorter workday. Previously when it was necessary for the majority of therapists to work extra hours to provide services to patients during a period with an unusually high census, I had no trouble staying late and working with more than my usual number of patients. After the stroke that would not be possible. Therefore, my supervisor further agreed that I would be allowed to arrive at a later hour in the mornings to avoid heavy commuter traffic. Arrangements were made for me to return to work in mid-September.

On a Monday morning in September of 1995, I stepped out of the elevator onto the second floor of the building, said good morning to the unit secretary, and then made my way down the hall leading to my office. Along the way I saw nurses and therapists with heads bent over patients' charts writing notes and reading physician's orders. I continued down the hall past the pediatric therapy gym toward my office. As I passed people on the way, they would say, "It's good to see you again," or, "Welcome back." I tried to meet their gazes and smile but found it difficult. My spontaneity of expression and responsiveness continued to be poor.

As I began to readjust to my work environment, it became obvious that the five-month break had distanced me from my work tasks. Getting back to work would not be easy, but I was determined to try. At first, I had been concerned that it would be extremely difficult for me to adjust to getting to work on time even at the later hour. In the beginning, it was especially strange to drive to work. In addition to the length of time that had elapsed, not being required to get myself anywhere on my own for most of the previous five months had made me less self-reliant than usual. Also, my initiation continued to be diminished and every activity required more than the usual time. My self-confidence was significantly lowered as well. During therapy, my cognitive rehabilitation therapist had suggested that driving an automatic transmission vehicle might present fewer difficulties than a standard transmission. I had always driven a standard transmission car and thinking about that kind of change was not particularly pleasant. After taking my driving evaluation, I felt that the therapist was correct. It was not an easy thing to resume driving with my lowered stamina and self-doubts.

After some discussion, Jerry and I agreed that it would be best to give up one of our standard transmission vehicles for an automatic one. When the time drew closer for me to return to work, we took his standard transmission Honda and traded it for an automatic transmission Mazda. Although it was a very nice car, I was not as comfortable with it as I had been with my own aging Nissan. Unlike pre-stroke days, there was little pleasure in my drive to work. Driving had always been one of my passions. I had always enjoyed driving my Nissan with a stick shift that made stops and starts so easy to control. Prior to my stroke, every driving experience had been pleasurable. Due to the stroke, those feelings were gone. In addition, I did not feel comfortable with music playing while I drove. It was a distraction that I felt I should avoid. In the past, I could not have imagined driving without listening to music. It was important that I fully readjust to driving. At the same time it was necessary to adjust to driving a new and different type of car. The impressive number of features in the car made for a certain level of possible confusion when it came to making adjustments to mirrors and such. The many buttons and lights on the dash were so different from my previous car. It made sense to me to reduce as many distractions as possible inside the car. There would be plenty of distraction on the outside to be dealt with. Although I did not know it then, adjusting to those changes would be the least of my problems after I got back to work.

Each day when I arrived at Genesis it was strange to see the same people that had treated me as therapists. This was not quite as strange as having it the other way around, but it was close. Getting back to communicating with fellow therapists and my supervisors felt unnatural and strenuous. My physical appearance had finally returned to mostly "normal" but I remained skeptical about how normal I looked to others.

Although I gradually became more comfortable driving the familiar route to work, I remained uneasy about my abilities. Having a shortened workday was beneficial, but it made me unhappy to require such a limited workday as compared to the past. Each day I went to work thankful to be able to return to the job I had enjoyed so much and hopeful that I would be capable of doing well. At the same time, I feared that I might be making a mistake by returning so soon (only five months) after the end of my therapy. Staying at home did not appear to be the best thing for me.

My supervisor had a good deal of experience with brain injury and stroke rehabilitation and she knew that it would be unrealistic to expect me to return to my job at the same level of productivity that existed before my stroke. In order to foster a positive transition, she adjusted my work schedule to the level of a newly hired therapist. Although that was helpful, there was no compensating for my loss of enthusiasm and cheerfulness that I had been known for prior to my stroke.

In 1990 when I had begun working, I had been given a probation period to become oriented to the hospital and the requirements of my particular position. During that period of probation, I spent time observing other therapists and reading various sources of information regarding treatment theory and practice, especially material related to neuropsychology. I had been very anxious to begin working with patients at that time, but thankful for the opportunity to learn from people who were more experienced than me. In my new situation returning after a stroke, I wanted to see patients. I was somewhat anxious, but less than I had been as a newly hired therapist. My concerns about my abilities caused me to welcome an opportunity to reacquaint myself with my work environment, materials, and methods.

My uneasiness was heightened by my perception that people were watching my every move in anticipation of some unusual behavior or expected failure. In addition, fellow therapists were curious about the possible cause of my stroke. On occasion, someone would ask, "Did they find out why it happened; was it stress?" I had trouble giving an answer. It surprised me that they would speculate that it was a matter of ill health. I'd shake my head and mutter, "It wasn't that kind of stroke." I was defensive about people thinking that I was unhealthy.

Although my responsibilities were far less than they had previously been, work was extremely taxing. I went to team meetings feeling poorly prepared and anxious about presenting data. Making progress reports in team conferences had always been a pleasant experience. Prior to the stroke, making critical judgments about patient progress had been very natural for me. It suddenly became a difficult and sometimes unclear task. In addition, it seemed that my previous familiarity with coworkers was replaced by a feeling of being in a group of strangers. My once lively delivery of reports no longer existed. Instead, it was stilted and dull. It seemed to me that some of my coworkers did not appreciate the full impact that my stroke had on me. In addition, it also appeared to me that they did not know how difficult it was for me to deal with the changes in my personality and my professional abilities.

I understood that they knew what they read in books and had seen in other patients, still, it was extremely difficult for me to cope with my perception that they didn't totally understand how my stroke had changed me. Perhaps some did not entirely understand the effects of a stroke on emotion or feelings. Additionally, my perception was that some coworkers didn't understand how emotion plays a part in a person's appearance and responses to other people. If your natural reactions are impacted by a stroke, relearning them does not come easily. I did not learn to speak or laugh spontaneously; it was always in me, like the color of my hair. Since that was the case, I had never learned to fake or create expressions. Maybe that was the reason that some coworkers seemed not to understand my loss of spontaneity and reflexive responses to jokes or to a question. During my time in outpatient therapy, the cognitive rehabilitation therapist worked with me on recognizing facial expressions and social cues and the speech therapist worked with me on vocal inflections and expressiveness. The damage to my right hemisphere, however, was too extensive and those functions could not be fully restored. That was not something I could explain to my fellow therapists in the course of a workday.

When I first returned to work people said, "You seem exactly the same." That made me confused. It was quite clear to me that I was not the same. It was, perhaps, a side effect of their having worked with me prior to my stroke and they were thinking of me as I was before rather than how I was afterward. It seemed to me that they didn't see the full effects that the stroke had on me. It worried me that they thought that I wasn't trying hard enough. My ability to show my feelings simply wasn't there. I sat in the meetings trying to pay close attention, but sometimes it was very hard. I sat there limp and lifeless without the expressiveness that they had previously seen in me. Before the stroke, my emotions were very strong. When I felt something I felt it all over. Whether it was a burst of pleasure at seeing a friend or the rush of embarrassment at a social blunder. Prior to my stroke, when I smiled at people it came from inside. When I had those feelings, other people could see them. At least I had believed they did.

Prior to the stroke when I had been having a particularly good day, I had been making a lot of progress with some things I was doing for a patient. I had accomplished a number of difficult tasks and was feeling particularly good. That day I stepped into an elevator and a man I didn't know was there. He looked at me and said, "You look like you just conquered the world." His remark made me smile. It also made me wonder, as usual, what he saw that caused him to make that statement.

After the stroke it was an entirely different situation. I did not have happy or sad feelings; I didn't have feelings about anything. I was listless and limp and barely responsive. I thought that I might just as well be bloodless. I wished I could express myself to people, but there seemed to be nothing I could do. I didn't laugh, I didn't cry, and I didn't smile very much. I didn't do those things because, even though I wanted to, I didn't seem to be able do them. Yet, people said, "You seem just the same." I think they were looking only at my physical appearance. I had no glaring physical disability, but my cognitive problems were not obvious to people. Still, some people would say that I was too expressionless and looked "miserable." Meanwhile, Jerry and I had to deal with changes in my behavior at home. My lack of enthusiasm extended beyond work. I frequently appeared to be very insensitive, and Jerry sometimes felt that I no longer cared for him. Also, the fatigue brought on by work was an additional interference with every aspect of our life together. Because I was I so physically tired, my mental functions became more slowed and dull. Every activity that required thought became incredibly difficult. My ability to process information was impaired by the fatigue making me less able to fully understand what was said to me. This was extremely frustrating for Jerry; he could become very short-tempered while trying to get a simple point across that seemed to be beyond my grasp. I would sometimes become defensive and that made things even worse. It seemed to him, however, that I did not care.

Another problem was that it became difficult for me to cope with Jerry being out of town for his job. In addition, he experienced more stress by trying to take care of me and keep up with his work responsibilities at the same time. Fortunately, while we experienced new, differently challenging problems, we remained as committed to each other as ever. The problems we encountered made it easy to see why marriages and other relationships break down when one partner has a stroke or acquires a brain injury from some other source.

As the end of September neared, it would be time to think about attending the annual Jacksonville Jazz Festival and to host the party we had each year prior to the festival itself. We talked a lot about the idea of not having the party since I was still adjusting to being back at work. It meant that time and energy were in short supply. I decided that the stroke had interrupted enough of my life and I wanted us to resume our normal activities as much as possible. In order to lessen interference with my work activity, we would work together on party plans only on weekends. We checked the calendar for suitable party dates and picked the Sunday prior to the festival. Having done that, we began developing a list of the CD's from festival performers that we wanted to buy. Although I felt that some people might criticize me for being concerned about having a party, I decided that what other people thought was not the most important thing. I wanted my life back and it seemed to me that it was time to be proactive about getting it. Things like parties might be viewed as insignificant when compared to issues like work or driving. In the context of returning to a normal life, doing something that you would normally do in spite of an interruption can be as valuable as work or any other activity. When I talked about the party at work, people said that they were surprised by my plans because they had assumed that we would not have the party.

Social activity and friendships are often compromised when a person experiences a stroke or other brain injury. I knew that it would be important for me to foster social relationships if they were to remain intact. More importantly, I felt that I needed to do things, like the party, that gave Jerry and me enjoyment. I did not intend to give up activities with friends that Jerry and I had made a part of our lives over the years.

At work I tried hard to keep up with my responsibilities. My inability to make changes in my style of interaction with other therapists was particularly disturbing. I hoped that people would understand that the stroke was still a factor rather than think that I did not enjoy being at work or that my feelings toward them had changed. There were times when I would find myself attempting to keep up with a discussion of patient progress or problems and find myself responding so slowly that I was certain everyone thought that it wasn't important to me. I might also find it difficult to maintain my attention as well as concentration.

Each day when I went home I would evaluate every action I had taken during the day in order to find possible problems. I felt very overwhelmed by what I had to do in my job, this was something unusual for me. It was impossible for me to see/know what I needed to fix so finding solutions became impossible.

Chapter 6—All That Jazz

Although issues at work continuously dominated my thoughts, Jerry and I made preparations for our annual Jacksonville Jazz Festival party in mid-September. I felt guilty about spending time making party plans when it was clear that work was more difficult to deal with than I had anticipated. Still, we both felt strongly about continuing to preserve the activities that had become integral to our friendships and general enjoyment of our lives. When we compiled the guest list, we had decided to continue our tradition of inviting people from both his and my work place. At first the idea of having any of my coworkers present was somewhat discomforting. In the end, we decided that it was best to maintain our tradition. In addition to that, we had talked during the summer about the idea that we should, after living together for 10 years, get married. With that in mind, we decided to make our party a combination Jazz Festival warm up and engagement announcement party.

The day of our Jazz Festival party the weather was clear and, because it was September, it was still pleasantly warm. We decided that it would be nice to take advantage of the remaining warm weather to enjoy the party outdoors on our deck. When we had begun making our plans for the party, I became worried about my ability to be a good hostess with all the requirements of that role. Fortunately, I knew that friends would offer to help out and make my job a little easier. That would not help me with my ability to be cheerful and peppy. In preparation for the party, Jerry went about finding champagne and getting needed accessories while I concentrated on food.

On the day of the party, we were uncharacteristically ready when the first doorbell rang. In a short time, couples and single people gathered in groups in the living room, the kitchen, and our deck. There was also a continuous stream of people moving between our house and our deck. The house became filled with sounds of music and happy voices. Eventually, conducting traffic and talking to people helped ease my self-consciousness. Still, I wondered about my appearance and responsiveness to our friends. I knew that there was a possibility that they would see me as remote and disinterested in them. There was no doubt that I would need to work to show my interest and pleasure at seeing them. Later, I would learn from a friend that my poor response to people had been interpreted as "cold."

Eventually everyone had migrated to the deck, so Jerry and I followed suit. I took a seat in the sun close to some friends that I had not seen for some time to enjoy pleasant conversation and catch up on any news they had about themselves. Jerry disappeared into the house but returned a few moments later with an easel. He set the easel up and called for everyone's attention. With some degree of flourish he placed a flip chart on the easel and "flipped" the pages until he came to a ten-item list. After he called everyone's attention to the list, he said, "Deborah and I have been together a while now and we think it's time for us to do something new." Some people were surprised and a few looked confused. Jerry went on to say, "We think it might _finally_ be O.K. for us to get married and here is our top ten list of reasons." One by one he went through the items on the list beginning at number 10 like David Letterman might do.

(10)   We both have dental insurance.

(9)   The homeowners association will be happier.

(8)   Lots of people already think we are.

(7)   Our mothers will be happier.

(6)   Newt (Gingrich) is getting rid of the marriage
       penalty tax (we hope).

(5)   It'll make introductions easier.

(4)   We already have a house and
       mortgage together.

(3)   We know each other pretty well since we have
       lived together for ten years.

(2)   We have a ring.

(1)   We want to!

After the list was completed and many nods of approval were over, he once again disappeared into the house. He returned with a box, from the box he took a bouquet of roses and placed them in my lap then he took out a small box. He opened the box and took out the ring that had been made for us. While holding the ring out toward me he asked, "Will you marry me?" Everyone applauded and I took the ring and said, "Yes." Then off he went again into the house, this time he returned with a jeroboam of champagne. He said he felt that a big event deserved a lot of champagne. There were toasts of congratulations, a number of jokes, and much time spent admiring the ring. I thought that it was good to be able to share the special occasion with our close friends, but I wondered if they could see that in my manner. I was sufficiently paranoid to think that my every move was being evaluated and judged. As I had anticipated, a few of my fellow therapists, including a few that had treated me as a patient, were present. I felt especially uncomfortable having them watch me. Each time I took a sip of champagne I worried that they were judging my actions.

As it grew late our guests departed. The house became quiet once again and we were feeling pleased with the turnout. Jerry was happy that his orchestration had gone so smoothly. I was impressed with his uncharacteristic calm while going through his presentation. He came up with the flip chart idea because his coworkers often teased him about his predisposition to use them during staff meetings. His proposal was not a spur of the moment act or unexpected. We had been discussing the idea of getting married since the summer. Our experiences during my hospitalization had given us reason to evaluate the limitations and problems that being unmarried presented. We had jokingly created the list of reasons. Our decision might have been prompted by some less than romantic ideas, but we knew it was important to consider practical issues related to our living arrangement. Although I was happy and felt good about the idea of getting married, I had a number of fears concerning the effects that my stroke might have on my abilities to keep up my responsibilities in our relationship.

We knew that getting married would not change the way we felt about each other, but I knew that my decreased abilities could have an adverse effect on our interactions. Some of our friends had said that they were pleased to see that we would finally "be official." Others wanted to know why we had not gotten married sooner. There was no straightforward answer to that. Sometime later, a friend of ours asked me, "What caused you to wait to get married, were you dating around and not sure?" I answered her, "I wasn't kissing frogs looking for a prince if that's what you mean."

She also asked me, "When you first met, why was it difficult for you to start seeing each other?" Then I explained to her that our decision about dating each other had been a difficult one because we had met under circumstances of a professional work association. She said, "Oh yeah, that can be really tough." She asked me several more questions about the situation. I explained to her that during the course of our normal work activities we had sometimes found ourselves dealing with a variety of problems related to my work at the ARC (Association for Retarded Citizens). Our interactions, for the most part, consisted of phone conversations regarding protocol and policy issues. Eventually though, Jerry asked me out. She asked, "What did you do for your first date?" I told her about our first date being on a sunny spring afternoon. I packed a picnic basket with boiled shrimp, French bread and a bottle of white wine. I picked him up after work at his office in downtown Pensacola then drove to Pensacola Beach. We sat on the beach and talked while we ate and afterward we walked in the surf for a while and talked some more. I drove him back to his car and we parted after making another date.

In the beginning I had been reluctant to get involved with him. He was a little older, more educated, and more accomplished than I, so I wondered why he wanted to get involved with me. After several dates, when he showed up at my door with a dozen roses, I was very suspicious about his motives. He told me later that he had wanted me to see that he was serious. After that day, we began seeing each other more regularly until it became exclusive. Over the course of a year or more we came to a mutual decision to live together. At first he had been concerned that it would not be acceptable to me. After multiple discussions, we agreed that we would give it a try. Also, we were both old enough to be logical and unhurried about something as serious as marriage. Additionally, we were both able to understand and respect each other's need to be cautious about something like getting married.

We also felt that if we decided to stay together, we would be prepared to make a decision about marriage under better circumstances. Due to my stroke, our circumstances hadn't exactly turned out to be better. We did have a very strong foundation for starting a marriage. We had no doubts about our feelings and we knew each other very well. We were best friends and very secure in our relationship. Still, I was worried that Jerry's motivation might be out a sense of obligation, and I didn't want it to be that way. The results of my stroke were a major source of concern. I knew that my behaviors did not match those of my pre-stroke self. I was uncertain about my ability to continue to be the kind of partner I had been in the past. This was especially clear given the problems we experienced after getting out of Genesis. Someone said something about our good fortune in being together. I said, "One very important factor in stroke recovery is a support system, so I'm more than a little fortunate." Almost any account of a stroke survivor will include a reference to a supportive spouse, family, or friends. For some people, it might be the most important part of a successful recovery from a stroke.

When everyone had gone, we cleaned up and sat down to talk about the Jazz Festival. The Jacksonville Jazz Festival would begin the following Thursday after our party and continue through Sunday. We checked the lineup of performers and decided to skip the days when the performers were those that we had seen more than once or twice. It turned out that we wanted to spend all of Saturday at the festival. I had no second thoughts or concerns about going. The Jazz Festival had become one of my favorite events.

The weather that Saturday turned out to be less pleasant for the festival than it had been for our party, but we had never allowed the weather to affect our attendance in the past. Umbrellas are not allowed during the festival so, as a rule, we always took rain ponchos as a precaution against the possibility of rain. Like most other people, we also took our beach chairs. We would usually arrive at the park very early in order to find a good spot close to the stage. That Saturday morning we got to the park around 10:00 a.m., a bit later than usual.

I was not in the least prepared for the effect that the music would have on me. I knew that my brain was still in the process of healing, but I did not realize that my emotional response functions were so far from being healed. As we made our way onto the grassy area in front of the stage, a performance was just beginning, and with the first musical notes, tears began to stream down my face in a torrent of emotion for which I was totally unprepared. Jerry was shocked and became upset wondering what had happened. I was just as shocked and confused by it as well. He did not understand that it was only the emotional lability that accompanies damage to the right hemisphere of the brain that caused me to lose my composure for no reason. He started asking me what was wrong, but when I tried to explain that there was no reason, it only made the situation worse. The more he questioned me the more I cried. Then suddenly it began to rain making the situation even worse. It seemed like there was nothing I could do to get myself together. Normally, such an event would not have occurred. With the emotional control system damaged it was not a simple matter to reestablish calm. It was necessary to let it run its course. Unfortunately, people were staring at us and that added to the mutual tension we were feeling. Also, I was unable to recognize that Jerry's reaction to the situation was confusion rather than anger. That was another result of the stroke.

The combination of rain and my inability to regain control over my emotional state made the situation intolerable, so we ended up abandoning our day at the festival. It was very disturbing to both of us and we went away feeling more confused and let down than at any other time in our relationship. Emotional control had always been one of my strong characteristics. Prior to the stroke, there were very few things serious enough to cause me to cry. In my position as a special education teacher and a cognitive rehabilitation therapist, emotional control had been particularly important. Therefore, it was understandable that my sudden loss of composure at the festival had confused Jerry and myself as well. Unfortunately, damage to my frontal lobes caused by the stroke had disabled the system that made it possible for me to exert control over my emotions. The system was still in the process of healing, but it would not be totally recovered for some time. Also, after the healing process was complete, there would be no guarantee that it would return to completely normal.

Until further healing could take place, it would be necessary to live with a maladjusted emotional system. I would cry for no reason at all, but not cry when there might be a reason. At the festival, Jerry became worried that he had done something to hurt me or that there was some problem that I had not told him about. When I explained to him that I did not know why it happened, it was difficult for him to accept. Thankfully, by the time we arrived home my emotional control had returned. We both felt a need to explore the problem, but I was distraught about the event and Jerry was having trouble dealing with it as well. There seemed to be no suitable approach to the subject. Although I knew that emotional lability from right hemisphere damage was the cause, I did not know why music had been the triggering event. After returning home from my discharge from therapy, I had noted a change in my response to music, but it had not been anything like the rush of emotion and sobbing that occurred at the festival. I had noticed that instead of the enjoyment that music usually gave me, there seemed to be nothing. It was as if music was reduced to nothing more than noise.

Appreciation of music is generally recognized as a right hemisphere function. Thus, the source of the problem was the stroke. Being aware of this was scary for me, but the situation had improved enough that I had felt comfortable about attending a live musical event. Unfortunately, the short span of time since the stroke was not enough for my more internal systems to be healed. While I had been in the hospital lability had surfaced, but not excessively. By the end of my outpatient program, things had been particularly stable. My emotional balance was askew in other less obvious ways, but on a day-to-day basis there had been no notable problems. The events at the Jazz Festival felt like a setback that left both of us confused and made me more worried about the prospects for continued healing and for the future in general. This was another reason for me to be concerned about our decision to get married.

After a week or two, I decided that I would begin to make plans for our marriage ceremony beginning in January. We began to talk about dates and decided that it might be possible to have the ceremony during November. Aside from setting a date, there were so many other things to be decided and many things to do to in preparation. I knew only the most basic elements of planning for a ceremony. I knew enough to recognize the level of difficulty of such an important event. The prospect of having to make arrangements and keep track of everything in the process was very intimidating. The first details like a dress and accessories could be dealt with in January. Everything else would have to wait until summer.

Later that year, we attended a Mary Chapin Carpenter concert. My emotional reaction to the concert was the same as when we had attended the Jazz Festival. That made me very discouraged about the improvement of my right hemisphere functions. Still, it seemed that avoiding concerts was not the best way to deal with the problem. Besides, live concerts had always been an enjoyable activity for me, and I did not intend to give them up due to emotional lability. I did not particularly like the idea that musical events or appreciation of music in general were impaired by the stroke. Who would welcome the loss of appreciation for music? I never want to lose the ability to enjoy music. How could it be okay not to enjoy those last two notes of "Steam Roller Blues?" Although not devastating, it was a dreadful thought. It was not reasonable to suddenly give up concerts or listening to music, but it was reasonable to assume that things would eventually improve.

Chapter 7—Lost in the Shuffle

Returning to work Monday, with memories of the Jazz Festival weekend, provoked a sense of unease. It was difficult for me to decide how much concern the episode might warrant. I knew I would need to find a reasonable solution to any similar issue that might arise. Unfortunately, how long that might take was anyone's guess. Nevertheless, I decided that it was best to focus fully on work.

Due to the requirements of my job, it eventually became necessary for me to take on more responsibility. Therefore, I resumed the use of methods developed over the years for keeping track of time and assignments. Although my true sense of time had always been poor, it was generally not an issue in day-to-day events at work. The stroke made the matter worse. A tight schedule and learning to use a "Day-Timer" system for keeping up with dates and deadlines had been very successful in the past. The stroke made it difficult for me to utilize the system well enough to keep me organized and timely. Also, my memory was less accurate than before, so note taking and reminder notes became much more important. Still, things like a loss of time tracking were more easily compensated for than less concrete or tangible processes such as judgment or decision making. On the other hand, if I was at home doing housekeeping tasks or cooking, time tracking problems were less problematic. If I forgot the pest control man's appointment, it was easier to deal with than forgetting an appointment with a patient's family member.

In addition to some general difficulties of readjustment to working, my positive feelings about being able to return to work were not in evidence on my face or in my manner of interactions with other people. My automatic emotional response system continued to be nonfunctional and it made me appear unreceptive or indifferent. Also, poor short-term memory made it difficult for me to accurately remember minor changes in the methodology of the regular patient assessments that were required. Familiar work methods and materials suddenly seemed strange to me.

Although I could remember my required activities and how to perform the tasks involved, a feeling of detachment left me uncertain about making judgements about patients. Historically, the ability to make quick and accurate assessments of people and situations had been one of my strengths. It was distressing to find that those skills were severely impacted by the stroke. I was fortunate to have a supervisor who made herself available to me if I needed her. Unfortunately, I began to feel that I might become a burden to her, so I was reticent about discussing issues with her.

In January of 1996 I began working a normal eight-hour day and running group therapy sessions in addition to individual ones. In the past this had presented no problems since I had a well-developed ability to do more than one thing at a time (multi-tasking). As a result of my stroke, that ability was significantly reduced. Problems began to surface in areas where there had previously been none. My supervisor had to remind me to be on time to meetings and that was unusual for me. Having her reassess my skills in accurately scoring patient evaluations was likewise unusual. That had also been an area of strength for me prior to my stroke.

Unlike my previous self, I became reluctant to seek feedback when I felt that I was not being given adequate information about my performance, or had an unclear understanding about my responsibilities. By March, it seemed that although I had finally returned to a normal workday, I was not working normally. On March 25, Jerry and I "celebrated" the one-year anniversary of my stroke. As always, the TPC Tournament was that week and we decided to attend as usual. In previous years we had taken advantage of our location close to the Marriott at Sawgrass where we could eat breakfast then take a ride on a "shuttle" boat that carried people across one of the many ponds near the golf course. The boat dropped us off at some point on the golf course, and we could catch up with the crowd or find one of the leaders to watch. We decided that we would take advantage of the services of the hotel that year so that the long walk from the TPC parking area to the course would not over tire me. I was glad that we had chosen not to miss the last day of the tournament so that we got to see Fred Couples win that year.

One year was a landmark that I had hoped would find me back at my former pace at work. That did not turn out to be the case. I was much less tolerant of minor difficulties. I also became less diligent about my behavior in the presence of other therapists or patients. It was not obvious to me that there was a problem with my motor planning ability until a day came when there was a tall man in a wheelchair with a broken leg fully extended in a cast. The courier had delivered him to my office, so at the end of our session I had to maneuver him out on my own. This was very difficult, but I tried to get him through the door without harm. We were stuck halfway in and halfway out of the door when a fellow therapist passed by. Just then my patience gave out, and I let out a good solid "Damn." This was definitely not professional behavior. I knew that the therapist had noted this and she would likely report it to my supervisor, but there was nothing to be done but apologize to the man and get him to his next therapy. After that experience my day improved a little, but it was a demoralizing episode. During my years as a teacher I developed a strong self-control appropriate to whatever a situation might require. I had known that there was a danger that my self-control might be compromised by the stroke, but I had believed, incorrectly, that it would be possible to recognize what was happening and thus be able to make corrections accordingly. Although I had feared that lability might resurface, that was not the specific problem that faced me. Instead, I was unable to accurately assess or adjust to various situations with coworkers or patients and I might behave inappropriately.

Another effect of the stroke was being easily frustrated by mistakes and heightened sensitivity to supervision. It was obvious that things were not the same as before the stroke, but if someone had asked me what the differences were, I would not have been able to tell them. No one asked me specific questions about work problems or needs but some people did ask things like, "How are you doing?" Since it was impossible for me to articulate my vague feelings of difficulty, I would always say, "Fine, I'm fine." The truth was that I was not fine. Work was harder than it had ever been in the past. I felt out of touch and uneasy most of the time. The things that I knew how to compensate for were not the things that would make a difference in my work. I had not forgotten or lost my knowledge but rather my ability to use my knowledge appropriately. Timeliness was an issue that could be kept under control by using aids like timers and schedules. It was more difficult to find a compensatory strategy for coping with my impatience, frustration, and feeling of detachment. Looking back, I can see many things that I could not see at the time. Although I understood the textbook explanations of the results of right hemisphere brain damage, it was difficult to reconcile the information with my personal experiences.

Multi-tasking, tracking time, and emotional control are higher executive functions generally attributed to the frontal lobes. My problems in these areas were caused by damage to the frontal lobes of my brain. When a blood clot lodged itself in the middle cerebral artery of my brain, cutting off blood flow to the major systems of the frontal lobes, my abilities were drastically altered. Prior to the stroke, my abilities in these areas had been very strong. During any part of my work schedule, I had previously able to keep track of the multiple pieces of information related to at least eight patients for individual therapy as well as group activities for up to ten patients. I had worked with a different patient every half-hour of my workday and facilitated two groups of patients every day for various periods ranging from one month to several months with a particular group of people. Those skills were the main reason that I was able to be good at my job. These most important and valuable aspects of my intuitive and intellectual abilities were eliminated with the death of the brain cells that made those skills possible. It was impossible for me to understand the problem, because the system in the frontal lobes that allowed me to know what was going on inside me was damaged. Although I wanted to understand the problem in order to correct it, there was no regulatory system functioning to allow me to do that.

In April of 1996 I was told that my performance was not up to standards and that it was necessary to put me on "administrative leave." Additionally, I was told there would be someone coming to perform a "fitness for duty" evaluation to determine whether it would be possible to reinstate me as a therapist. This made me extremely unhappy and distressed, but I knew that it was out of my hands at that point. On May 1, Jerry and I celebrated our 11th year anniversary of being a couple. This one would be at home with each of us feeling the strain of my work difficulties.

On May 17, the same neuropsychologist that had conducted my neuropsychological exam the previous summer came to Genesis to make a fitness for duty evaluation. After reviewing my paperwork related to the therapy activities with my patients, as well as documentation from my supervisor regarding the problems that she had observed, the neuropsychologist interviewed my supervisor and me. Each of us was asked about our perceptions of my daily work activities in order to determine the extent of my problems. In one interview session, I became especially frustrated with the question, "Why do you want to work?" I wanted to scream, "How dare you question my motivation for continuing to work in my profession!" All I could do was sit there in mute silence. In the past I might not have spoken either, but I probably would have given a look that could singe someone's eyebrows. Unfortunately, I could not do that either. In retrospect, I understand why the question was asked, but at the time it was difficult to appreciate its value.

On the 23rd of May, the fitness for duty report was delivered to Genesis and my supervisor gave me a copy to review. The report described the problems that were evident in my ability to work as a therapist. In the report, problems were noted related to organization, planning, problem solving, critical thinking, and multiple tasking. These problems were in areas which are very typical of right hemisphere brain damage. These right hemisphere skills are critical for a therapist or teacher. It was noted that although I had some sense of my problems, I was unable to correct them. The report further indicated that I was not able to perform a large number of the most important functions in my job description. Perhaps worst of all, these continued cognitive problems could possibly compromise my treatment of my patients. This information was so tremendously different from any evaluation that I had ever had in the past. Previously many words had been used to describe my capabilities as an employee, among them: thorough, precise, competent, and an asset, but never incapable. In all of my previous work history, no one ever said that I was not capable of performing any and all duties necessary for my job. This was a crushing blow to my self-esteem and belief in myself. It was clear that I suddenly became incompetent because of an unforeseeable event. I could not imagine what I would do. I had always believed that I could return to work. There, however, in black and white was the recommendation that I be placed on total disability because I could not perform the duties of my position as a cognitive therapist or a job of any kind.

Chapter 8—Insult to Injury

Allison, my longtime friend and co-worker, handed me her car keys and said, "I've got to return this equipment, then I'll catch up with you." We were in the Health Science's Building at the University of North Florida where she was enrolled in a Master's degree program and had asked me to help her with a class project. Allison was one person who had maintained contact with me after I lost my job. When she asked me to help her with her project, it was easy to agree. Although I was able to drive, it continued to be a problem. Trips to the grocery store and other short distances were okay with Jerry, but he was uncomfortable with any other distances. Therefore, when Allison asked me to participate in her project, we had decided that it was easier for her to do the driving.

I took the keys from her and stepped out of the door of the building and made my way toward the trees where she had parked her car. It was Wednesday, July 3, 1996 and a clear summer day. On our way to the University we had talked about possible Fourth of July activities and told each other stories about past Fourth of July experiences. We both had stories of good, bad, and embarrassing Fourth of July experiences.

Before I could get to the car, one continuous repetitive sound, like a lone rhythmic drumbeat or one guitar string being plucked, sounded in my ears. It gradually became louder and louder until it was all I could hear. Suddenly, I realized that it was not an environmental sound, but one that was inside my own head. At the same time, I was gripped with an unbelievable fear, and I could barely hold the car keys. Allison had not caught up with me by the time I had reached the car. I wanted to get into the car as soon as possible to wait for her, but I could not seem to get the key into the lock. I had no idea what the noise was about, and I was frightened. It seemed certain that whatever it might be, it couldn't be anything good. Finally, Allison arrived; shakily, I handed her the keys and we both got into the car. She immediately knew that something was wrong and she asked me, "What's wrong?" All I could tell her was that I was hearing a strange loud noise, and I was very scared. It was mid-afternoon so Jerry, naturally, was at work. His office was only minutes from the University so we were closer to him than to our house.

Neither of us knew what might be happening, and she said she did not feel comfortable about taking me home and leaving me alone. After very little discussion, we both decided it might be a good idea to go to Jerry's office. I tried to relax and hoped that the noise would go away. After a few minutes the sound began to diminish, so I was hopeful that it was nothing serious. By the time we got to Jerry's office, I was feeling a little better. Suddenly I discovered that my left arm was numb.

It was as if all the circulation had been cut off starting at my left shoulder. The only good thing was that it felt like the numbness of blood restriction rather than the paresis of a stroke. Still, the three of us became worried by this new development. Jerry made the suggestion that we should go to the hospital. I couldn't argue with the idea so we decided to go to the emergency room immediately. When we arrived at the hospital, we were told we would have to wait to be checked in. My arm did not feel any better, but my fear had somewhat subsided. My head was only beginning to get quiet. It seemed as if I was in a surrealistic dream. Our wait continued for some time while we remained anxious about the situation. Anyone who is unfortunate enough to need emergency room services may not feel that their emergency is being seen as an emergency. All the urgency is an undercurrent that we do not see until it is our turn to have our needs dealt with. Eventually a nurse came to show us to an examination room. I sat on the large examination chaise as she had directed me to do while waiting for my neurologist to arrive. Fortunately, Jerry and Allison remained with me.

A few minutes later, a nurse arrived and said that the neurologist had been called and that some tests were needed before he arrived. At this point we had not seen a physician. Suddenly, my left leg began to shake, then my left arm contracted upward as if to punch me in the face. Then there was nothing but darkness. I woke up looking at the ceiling of the exam room barely able to move with no memory of what had happened. My limbs responded, but very slowly. I could see, but the picture was a little fuzzy. My head hurt and there was a humming quality to it. A doctor was there, but I didn't remember seeing him enter the room. Since my neurologist was not on duty that day, the neurologist on call had come in to make an assessment. After his assessment was completed, I was put into a wheelchair and taken to another room for an EEG (electroencephalogram). I remember getting into the wheelchair but not the test itself.

The EEG confirmed the existence of abnormal electrical activity in my brain. Apparently, scar tissue on my temporal lobe left by the stroke had created an abnormal area of brain activity that resulted in a seizure. Afterward, the neurologist told me that I was not having another stroke, but that I had experienced a grand mal seizure. He then told us that it was necessary to prevent further seizure activity. To do that, he ordered an anticonvulsant medication to be given intravenously (IV). I was hooked up once more to a buzzing, whirring machine that dispensed medication into my system in order to calm my brain and prevent any further seizure activity. Later, when my regular neurologist arrived, he told us that he wanted to admit me to the hospital. He also told us that the noise I had heard was an "aura," the result of the initial abnormal brain activity that signals the onset of a seizure. The numbness in my arm was also part of the aura phase of the seizure. The auditory and sensory aura was the result of damage in specific areas of my brain, most likely the temporal and parietal lobes. Because I had not experienced any seizure activity previously, I did not know this was the case. For what seemed like a very long time after the seizure, I was so weak that I could barely stand. This is very typical after a convulsive seizure. Every muscle in my body was totally depleted of strength. It was a relief to get into a bed. I went to sleep that night with the IV in my arm not knowing what the next day would bring.

The next day I was relieved to again see my regular neurologist. He came to tell me that I had a seizure disorder, but that I did not have epilepsy. The distinction between the two is that epilepsy is a condition with a tendency to have recurring seizures. Posttraumatic seizures are the same in nature as epilepsy but may not be recurring. The type of seizure I had experienced was Grand Mal or Tonic-Clonic. These are convulsive seizures with abnormal electrical (neuronal activity), beginning in a small part of the brain and quickly spreading to the adjoining parts of the brain until the entire area has abnormal electrical activity. The chaotic nature of the electrical activity usually results in a temporary loss of consciousness along with severe muscle spasms and jerking throughout the body. A postictal (post-seizure) state is most common after convulsive seizures such as grand mal. It may include headache, temporary confusion, and being fatigued. All of those things were apparent in my postictal state. Generally, a person does not even remember the seizure event itself. This was also the case with me.

It was very difficult to be relaxed about being admitted to the hospital. Yet, hospitalization proved to be the easiest aspect of dealing with my seizure disorder. Thankfully, I spent an uneventful Wednesday and Thursday in the ICU. I was discharged on Friday, July 5. At that time, I was given an oral anticonvulsant medication before leaving the hospital. I was instructed to make an appointment to see my neurologist as soon as possible. Although it was a relief to be able to go home, I was anxious about the possibility of another seizure.

Something that reinforced that feeling was noise. After the stroke I began hearing constant noise in my head. The sound of bells, whistles, humming, whirring, and numerous other things kept me awake at night, and made it difficult for me to hear or to think clearly. After the seizure the sounds seemed to be not only more intense, but of a greater variety as well. I heard the doorbell ring when there was no one there or the telephone when it wasn't ringing.

After learning that the sound I'd heard in the parking lot had been the precursor to a seizure, I became more sensitive and aware of the existing noises in my head. In addition to those problems, I was prohibited from driving due to the seizure. I had been so glad to be able to return to driving after being restricted from it by the stroke. I was heartsick to be restricted from it once again. Knowing that there was a chance that my brain might suddenly go haywire resulting in a seizure made me feel less inclined toward driving in spite of any distress at losing my privilege. If I could not feel safe in my house, I certainly didn't want to be out on the road. Also, I did not know what had occurred during the seizure. That made me insecure about being alone. I did not know whether there would always be an aura before a seizure. I did know that a seizure can happen very suddenly and a resulting fall could be very serious. This made me so nervous that I couldn't take a shower comfortably unless Jerry was at least in the house, if not in the same room. That was something that had to change very quickly since he would always be off to work much earlier than I would rise.

Thankfully, after a few weeks I was able to develop some confidence in the idea that my medication would prevent any seizure activity. I remained uneasy about the situation, nonetheless. The first few days were the worst. I found it difficult not to think about the possibility of having a seizure. Fortunately, Jerry's office was close enough that he would be able to get home in the event of an emergency. In order to help us both worry less about the problem, we developed a plan for dealing with any seizure situation. First of all, I hoped that an aura would give me a few minutes to get to some place of relative safety. The first thing we did was to program Jerry's work number into the phone. In the event that he was not in his office or the line was busy, I could call his pager number, also programmed into the phone. If I knew or thought that a seizure was eminent, we had a twofold plan. First, I would make sure I got to a safe place, like the bed. Then I would call or page him to let him know that I might need him to come home. If I had to page him, he would try to call me immediately to see if I was able to answer the phone. The next course of action was dependent upon whether or not I answered the phone.

In addition to this plan, I had the advantage of good neighbors to help me if Jerry was unable to get in touch with me or get to me. The phone numbers of two neighbors were also programmed into the phone in the event that it might be necessary to contact one of them for assistance. Depending on my memory or having an ability to think fast enough to get help was not particularly wise.

With a strategy worked out to deal with the situation, we were able to feel more relaxed. Thankfully, I did not have another seizure and after a while it seemed evident that the medication was working. In spite of that, I periodically experienced auras. The aura would generally dissipate without developing into a seizure, but there was no way to know when it would fade away or when it would become a seizure. I learned to deal with that by using some relaxation exercises. On a few occasions, I would go to my neighbor to talk to her while I waited for the aura to cease or as a precaution should a seizure occur. Auras happened most often at about 2 a.m. This would jolt me out of a sound sleep. Fortunately, they would not last more than a few minutes. The situation kept me in a constant state of unease. This issue further complicated my being at home alone every day.

Anticonvulsant medication comes with a myriad assortment of problems, including the continuous need to monitor blood serum levels, and numerous possible side effects. The medication must reach a particular level in the bloodstream in order to be effective. At the same time, it cannot be too high or it may become toxic. These levels must be monitored through blood tests on a regular basis in order to assure a proper amount of medication is in the blood so that a person will not be under or over medicated.

Unfortunately, it is difficult to be absolutely certain that a particular drug will work to inhibit seizure activity in any individual. What may be therapeutic for one person may not be therapeutic for another. Also, one particular drug may not work for some people the way it does for others. Some people may require two different medications in combination. Anticonvulsant medications are typically chosen based upon the type of seizure. Different drugs work for different seizure types. My neurologist first decided to prescribe Tegretol. He explained that the nature of my disorder was focal (specific) rather than diffuse (general). Tegretol is generally recognized as a drug that can effectively control focal (Tonic-Clonic) seizure activity. Thankfully, I was free of seizures for the remainder of the summer.

Each week Jerry drove me to the lab for bloodwork in order to allow my neurologist to make judgements about my medication doses. Unfortunately, the aura problem continued to be an issue and the neurologist wanted to change my medication to try to correct it. In the fall he began the process of transition from Tegretol to a relatively new drug called Lamotrigine (Lamictal). The transition would take several weeks and possibly longer to achieve a proper level for controlling seizure activity. It was necessary to gradually decrease the Tegretol dose while slowly adding the Lamotrigine. My neurologist said that he hoped that I would eventually take only the Lamotrigine.

During the transition period for this process, I was very nervous about the possibility of a seizure. The new drug would not be at a therapeutic level for some time, and I was worried that as one was decreased the other would not be enough. My fears were validated when the seizure aura continued to occur from time to time. Fortunately, the neurologist was very sympathetic to my concerns and was always available for advice when I needed it. The continuous need for lab work was another unpleasant aspect of the situation. If that were not enough, problems with medical insurance payments and billing errors kept me busy troubleshooting. Jerry said one day, "It's a good thing you're not working." Then I had to say, "If I was working I would not need these services." While I dealt with these issues, there were the ongoing preparations for the marriage ceremony to take care of as well. I felt that it would be a miracle if I got anything accomplished at all. Eventually, after Lamotrigine was my only medication, it was necessary to make adjustments in the doses several times in order to stop the auras that had continued to plague me. It was sometimes difficult to keep track of a complicated schedule like one pill every three days or alternating one and two pills every three days respectively. It seemed like the seizure disorder was a full time job.

Eventually, my neurologist decided that the best way to deal with the auras was to add a second medication. The medication he chose to add to the Lamotrigine was Dilantin. After a few weeks with the combination of Lamotrigine and Dilantin, the auras finally ceased. After weeks of problems with a seizure aura every night, I could finally get a full night's sleep again. The blood serum levels were tested weekly until it seemed that the levels were stable. After a while when the levels appeared to be stable, the monitoring schedule was adjusted to every two weeks. Unfortunately, the nature of some medications can result in fluctuations in blood serum levels without notice until the levels are too low to be effective or too high. Slowly the serum levels can rise steadily until a state of toxicity occurs. Toxicity is a serious issue.

In the fall, my Dilantin serum level dropped below the therapeutic level and seizure auras returned. The neurologist became concerned that the level might be low enough to allow seizure activity. Therefore, he increased the Dilantin dosage until the range became therapeutic again. For some reason the level began to rise significantly in my system. I became lethargic and unsteady on my feet. I also developed perfectly clear double vision. Eventually, I was walking like an extremely drunken person. The double vision became more severe over time and the combination of those conditions created a potential for serious harm. One weekend, Jerry and I left for Pensacola, where he was to attend a meeting the following week. In the interest of safety, Jerry made me go with him on the trip. We left on Friday, and on the way we decided to stop in Tallahassee to reduce the fatigue of the trip. By that time, I was so unsteady on my feet that it was unsafe for me to go anywhere alone. On Saturday afternoon, to prevent total boredom, we decided to go to a large mall. When we got there my ability to walk in a straight line was completely gone. We had no choice but to leave the mall and return to our hotel. Jerry decided that the only thing to do was get in touch with my neurologist to appraise him of the situation.

After the neurologist heard his explanation of my condition, he told us to get a STAT blood serum level. That sounded easy enough but it turned out to be a complicated activity. We could not find a doctor who would agree to take a blood sample in his office. Therefore, we had to find an emergency room instead. By the time we got to an emergency room, it was well after dark. Thankfully, my neurologist was able to fax a lab order to the emergency room doctor very quickly and my blood was tested. The attending physician came to tell me the results of the test. He told us what we already knew: my serum level was toxic. He told me to stop taking the Dilantin for three days starting that evening. That made me nervous. I asked him if it was really okay to stop taking it suddenly. He looked at me seriously and, clenching his fist, he said,

"If you don't, your heart will stop." That changed the situation considerably. Dilantin has a half-life of about three days, so not taking it would have no adverse effect on me. I followed his orders and within a week I was back to a normal walk again. I also went to see my neurologist as soon as it was possible.

Unfortunately, that would not be the last of my troubles with seizure medication. When the neurologist saw me after the toxic episode, he mapped out a plan to try to keep the Dilantin level stable. The resulting dose schedule was very complicated. The dosing schedule called for alternating numbers of pills as well as alternating pill strengths. After several more weeks of constant monitoring, the level finally seemed to stabilize. That was not as reassuring as it might sound.

Once, during an interview with a mental health counselor, I was asked about my seizure disorder and its effect on my day-to-day functioning. I was very honest in telling him that the situation was a source of stress. After we talked for a while about the seizures, I confided to him about my continuous problems with attention and concentration as well as concerns about experiencing seizures. He shrugged his shoulders and said, "So, I know people that have a lot of seizures during one day." Still, I had no previous experience with seizure activity and it was very difficult to adjust to the situation. Also, it was a glaring reminder of the damage to my brain that was caused by the stroke.

Chapter 9—The House on Bayou Road

At the time that Jerry and I finally decided on a date for getting married, we remained undecided about the choice of a location. We thought that it would be fun to go out of state. We talked at first about going to California but after some research, we decided that we would have the ceremony in some other place and spend our honeymoon in California.

One of our earliest dates, long before the ravages of Hurricane Katrina, had been a trip to New Orleans for Sunday brunch at the Windsor Court Hotel. After that, New Orleans became one of our favorite places to visit. We would drive from Pensacola to New Orleans on a Sunday morning and spend just the day, or on a Friday afternoon and spend the weekend, drive back to Pensacola in the afternoon or the next day, respectively. At the time we were to be married, one of my sisters was living close to New Orleans. After some discussion, we determined that we would explore the possibility of having the ceremony in New Orleans. We found that New Orleans had many places that were suitable for such occasions. Ours would not be a wedding in a conventional sense. I told Jerry that we had always been unconventional, and I could see no reason to change that. We were not young people just starting a life together. Still, we wanted to do something special.

One afternoon, while looking through some travel guides for New Orleans, we found what we were looking for. It was a place that would be quiet, romantic, and receptive to our needs. It was a "Petite Creole" plantation that had become a bed and breakfast or inn. The House on Bayou Road was located off Esplanade Ave. between the French Quarter and the New Orleans Museum of Art. From the inn's information pamphlet, I learned that in 1798 Domino Fleitas, a physician/diplomat from Tenerife in the Canary Islands, built the home as the main house to an Indigo Plantation. The house was built in the West Indies Creole style with wide galleries and many French doors opening onto flowering patios. In the spring of 1996, we took a trip to New Orleans to take a look at the place before making a commitment. As soon as we saw it we knew it would be an excellent place for our ceremony. In addition to the main house, a private cottage complete with a four-poster bed, beamed ceilings and a fireplace as well as a porch with rocking chairs sat on the edge of the garden. There was also a pool near the main house. With all the amenities it offered, we concluded that it was perfect.

We wanted to start making plans as soon as we returned to Ponte Vedra Beach, knowing that it would take some time to make arrangements to be married in a different state. It would be necessary to start as soon as possible. We had decided early in our discussions to have the ceremony in November. We consulted calendars for specific dates, and Jerry looked at his work obligations to avoid conflicts. The best time turned out to be the week of Thanksgiving. The Friday after Thanksgiving was the 29th. We decided to have our ceremony on that date. Our first task would be to learn the laws in the State of Louisiana concerning marriages, as well as the process of getting a license. Jerry set about searching the internet for the information we needed. After many phone calls over the course of two weeks, we had made reservations for our stay, and other arrangements. Also, Jerry had obtained all the necessary information about getting a license and had engaged a local judge to perform the ceremony. In the beginning, I had been very nervous about being able to properly make all the necessary arrangements. Everything had to be done correctly or we might not have a ceremony. I didn't know very much about planning a wedding. Still, I figured that it wasn't necessary to be a rocket scientist to plan a straightforward marriage ceremony. At the same time, I knew that there were many details involved. I was afraid that my cognitive problems would interfere with my ability to make the arrangements properly. I also knew that my lack of experience with wedding planning might be a disadvantage. Therefore, I looked for inspiration as well as information in various resources about weddings. Bridal magazines and Idiot's Guides became part of my wedding research library. It was important that nothing was forgotten. Lists of every possible aspect of a wedding littered the coffee table on a daily basis. I made lists for everything and post-it notes marked pages in books and magazines.

Unfortunately, my organization tended to run into disorganization. The problems that had confronted me at work were also evident in my efforts to plan our marriage ceremony. There were enough resources to provide ample information but it frequently seemed that pages in books or magazines were marked and then placed out of the way. Thus, they were forgotten and this made retrieving the information extremely difficult as well as frustrating. Also, it seemed there was so much information in my head that I could not keep track of most of it.

Since we were going out of state, we decided not to ask people to make a trip to the ceremony. We chose to have a small family-only ceremony and to have a big party to celebrate with our friends back in Ponte Vedra Beach at a later date. This would be a delayed "wedding reception" after we returned from our trip to California and were sufficiently recovered from all the travel. Accordingly, we ordered wedding announcements instead of wedding invitations. The choices for wedding announcements was somewhat overwhelming and it was difficult to find something we both liked, but after viewing selections from several companies, we found what we wanted. After about a month of constant work, the arrangements were finalized. One item that had to be dealt with at home was pictures. We found a local photographer to take still shots to use in newspaper announcements and such. When we went to sit for the pictures, it was difficult not to think about the asymmetry of my face. My fears were somewhat confirmed when the photographer asked, "Is that your normal smile?" Thankfully, we were able to get enough good shots to use. We knew we would take many more pictures at the time of the ceremony.

After all the arrangements for our stay at the Inn and for the ceremony, there remained the issue of family to be dealt with. Most of Jerry's family was in Arizona. His father was deceased and his mother had been in ill health for some time. It was not realistic to expect her to make the trip. My family, on the other hand, was closer. My father was also deceased, but my mother was still in good health and living near Pensacola. My sister, Linda, lived close to New Orleans in the town of Slidell. She graciously invited all the family to her house for Thanksgiving dinner. That meant that all my sisters and my mother would have a perfect reason to be close to New Orleans the week of Thanksgiving. I talked with Linda about a crazy idea I had to make the wedding a surprise for my mother and two sisters who lived in Northwest Florida. We decided that it would eliminate a lot of anxiety for everyone involved. Linda had done a great job of planning her own wedding, so she became my main source of not only information but guidance as well. We conspired together about my surprise wedding well in advance so that our plans would remain a surprise. I also had many talks with her about the arrangements in order to improve the chances that nothing would be forgotten.

By November I was confident that the ceremony would go smoothly and that we would have a nice surprise for everyone. When the time came, we would travel to Slidell to spend a few days visiting with my family until Thanksgiving was over. We planned to give everyone a good reason to stay over in Slidell by saying we would go out in New Orleans on a tour and have dinner somewhere on Bourbon Street. The day after Thanksgiving would be the day we would marry, so we wanted to be rested and relaxed. I had finally begun to feel confident that my seizure medication was working, since I had not experienced a seizure since the first one in the summer of 1995. I was feeling confident that I would be able to enjoy my activities worry free.

We set out for Louisiana the morning of Saturday the 23rd and arrived late that afternoon. We spent that evening with my sister and her family. On Sunday, Jerry and I traveled into New Orleans just to stroll around town. We also took advantage of the opportunity to dine in some restaurants we had not visited on previous trips. On Monday we were back in New Orleans to get our marriage license. In the evening my sister and I enjoyed visiting together and going over plans for the ceremony. She cooked dinner for us, and afterward she and I sat talking over the remains of a bottle of wine. I had not been drinking much due to the limitations placed on me by the seizure disorder and anticonvulsant medication. We did not see each other often due to our geographical separation so getting to talk together was a welcome treat. We were both well aware of the problems associated with too much drinking, so we held to our decision to limit our intake.

Early the next morning, I woke very suddenly to the sound of a seizure aura pounding in my head. Although there was no numbness in my arm, I knew immediately that it would progress into a seizure. Jerry helped me out of bed and walked me to the kitchen reassuring me on the way. Linda was on a break from work for the holiday, and she was in the kitchen getting ready to make breakfast for everyone. The three of us sat at the kitchen table and talked for a few minutes. Suddenly, my body slumped forward and I was shaking all over as a seizure began. Jerry and Linda managed to get me onto the floor, since it seemed clear that I would not be able to remain in the chair. Unlike the first seizure, I remained conscious and somewhat aware of the shaking and spasms of my body. I was unable to respond or communicate in any way, but I knew what was happening. I could hear and see, but not clearly. The muscle spasms jerked and twisted my body like wringing out a washcloth. The seizure lasted only minutes, but felt like a very long time. When it was over, I felt greatly relieved, but extremely tired. The after effects did not seem to be as severe as my initial seizure, but I needed help to walk and had a very bad headache. Jerry helped me back into bed to rest; Linda gave me a bell to ring for help in the event that seizure activity was to resume. Mercifully, there were no further problems related to seizures the remainder of the day. Unfortunately, my peace of mind was destroyed. As my strength slowly returned, we all began to relax.

Fortunately, we were able to contact my neurologist back in Jacksonville to inform him of the event and to get his advice regarding anything we should do. It was difficult to make a definite conclusion about the possible cause of the seizure because there were variables other than the wine involved. One of the variables was an antihistamine that I had been taking for several years. My neurologist advised us to go to a doctor as soon as we were able. We found a physician in Slidell, so we went to the doctor late Tuesday afternoon. After seeing the doctor, there was little to be done at that time except to stop taking my antihistamine. Because there was a degree of uncertainty about the cause of the seizure, I was left in a state of apprehension for the remainder of our stay in New Orleans. My mother and my other two sisters arrived for their Thanksgiving visit, and somehow we were able to continue to keep our plans a secret. We had a lot of food for our Thanksgiving dinner, but there was some tension in the air, as everyone, myself included, seemed to be worried that I would have a seizure at any given moment. I was very self-conscious and overly sensitive to the situation as well. Thanks to Linda things went very smoothly. We enjoyed traditional as well as less than traditional fare along with a few Creole dishes she had prepared. We reluctantly eliminated wine but that did not detract from our enjoyment.

On Friday morning, Jerry and I went to The House on Bayou Road to check in and make preparations. The ceremony would take place in the private cottage at 2:00 p.m. on Saturday. My sister Linda and her husband Mark were the first to arrive that day, followed closely by my mother and two other sisters. Linda had told my mother and sisters that they were in for a special lunch at a plantation. While I hid in the bathroom of the cottage, Linda and her husband, Mark, greeted everyone at the door. When my mother saw the decorations in the cottage and noted Linda and Mark's attire she asked, "Is this what I think it is?" Linda told her that it was, then got everyone appropriately situated inside and we waited for the judge to arrive. While we waited for the time of the ceremony, it was impossible not to worry about the possibility of another seizure. Eventually it had to be put out of my mind or it would intrude on my concentration during the ceremony. A few minutes before the scheduled time, the judge had not arrived and we were nervous that there might be a problem. A few minutes after 2:00 p.m. the judge came to the door and explained that he had mistakenly been in the main house waiting for us. We welcomed him into the cottage and wasted no time getting on with the formalities. Things went very smoothly afterward. Although it was not a large formal affair with a lot of people and a long aisle to walk down to the sound of the wedding march, it was a lovely and pleasant event.

There was only one small incident during the ceremony itself. I have come to believe that there is some unwritten rule that every wedding ceremony must have at least one small blooper. In any wedding I have attended there has always been one. Once a friend's father stood on her long veil while she attempted to enter the church. A nervous groom dropped the ring in another. My sister and brother-in-law had been unable to light the candle in their ceremony and there were other bloopers that I had witnessed. For mine, there was Jerry saying "my lawfully leaded wife." It was difficult not to laugh, but we ignored it and kept going. When the ceremony was over we stepped outside to make our way to the main house for some traditional Creole food prepared by the house chef. When we opened the door, we encountered a misty rain. We made our way to the main house and spent a leisurely time eating red beans and rice, as well as gumbo and making toasts. We had my favorite champagne, Veuve Clicquot, but I could not relax enough to drink any of it. Instead, I drank some non-alcoholic champagne we had brought along. We had a few toasts before cutting the cake , then we danced until everyone had to leave for home. Jerry and I stayed in the cottage that night. We planned to pack up and head to the airport the next day to start our trip to California. Our trip would begin with a stop in San Francisco for 2 –3 days and then on to the wine producing areas of Napa and Sonoma.

This would not be our first or last trip to the wine country; therefore, we planned to see places that we had missed on our previous trips. Those experiences gave us the advantage of knowing where we wanted to go and when. It also gave us a good idea about how to deal with the possibility of over-consumption of wine in the process of exploring the offerings of various wineries. After my experience in New Orleans there was little doubt that I would be extremely cautious about drinking. The time of year would also make it a little less hectic. Our flight was uneventful, but when we got off the plane in San Francisco, we noticed the chill in the air. Fortunately, we were prepared for the difference in the weather. We followed our plans to get a rental car and proceeded into the city to find our hotel. We were pleased to find that it was a very quaint hotel within walking distance of a few places we wanted to see. We walked around the immediate area the next day and discovered that we were not accustomed to walking up and down so many hills. Still, we were not deterred and enjoyed the sights and every aspect of our visit.

On Monday we set out for Napa Valley. We had reservations at a bed and breakfast inn within easy driving distance of many vineyards. We spent the weekdays driving from one place to another to enjoy the scenery and do some wine tasting. A positive side effect of my limit on consumption allowed me to be more selective in choosing wines to taste. We knew it would be impossible to see everything we had missed on previous trips, but we set out to see as much as we could. In spite of the time of year, we were pleasantly surprised that we were not freezing every day. Each winery that we visited had warm, comfortable tasting rooms and we had very enjoyable visits. By the end of our two weeks we were tired and ready to head home. Thankfully, we managed to make it through our entire stay without any problems related to my seizure disorder. The only problem we encountered involved the baseball caps, wine glasses, and t-shirts that we collected on our visits to the various wineries. They needed separate luggage.

We returned home tired, but happy. As soon as the holidays were over it would be time to plan our belated "reception party." It seemed that the party might be a bigger challenge than the ceremony. Sending the invitations would be easy because they could be included with our announcement. The ordeal of preparing and mailing invitations or announcements was a challenge for me. Nevertheless, it was possible to get the announcements and party invitations properly addressed and placed in each envelope with less difficulty than I had anticipated. Fortunately, Jerry helped with making the list of names and addresses. He was too busy getting back into work after being gone, so it was not possible for him to help with the actual writing of names on the party invitation envelopes or to address the announcement envelopes. Jerry did take time to check everything to find any mistakes that I might have made. By some miracle, there were very few mistakes. There were, of course, a few envelopes that had to be thrown out because of one error or another. In general, the process went well. One problem was making certain that people's names were spelled correctly and that addresses were clearly written and in the proper position on the envelope. It could be very disappointing to find that an envelope had been addressed upside down or incorrectly addressed. Another problem was my handwriting. It was very difficult to keep it clear and legible.

We had set the date for our party in mid-January in hopes that people would be recovered from Christmas and New Year's celebrations. For the party, the food was a combination of catered and my own creations. I decided to get a large simple sheet cake just for fun. It turned out to be a beautiful day for our celebration. Nearly everyone we invited came. It was surprising to me how generous our friends were with gifts. Since we were not exactly newlyweds in need of basic household items, people were very creative. It made us feel fortunate to have so many good friends to celebrate our marriage. I was able to be only minimally concerned about my appearance. There were so many things to keep me busy. That made it possible for me to concentrate on my actions instead. We had so much fun, it was a letdown when it was over. Still, we knew there would be more times for us to get together with many of our friends for other occasions. Afterward, it was good to see that things went so well, and yet it was difficult to put fears about making people see me as cold or insensitive out of my mind.

Chapter 10—Better, But Not the Same

After the California trip and reception party were over, it was time to get back to normal. While that meant that Jerry would go back to his regular work routine, I would be making the adjustment to being a housewife. This was new territory for me. I had been working since college and it was very strange to see Jerry go off to work and for me to stay at home. Although I continued to struggle to take care of myself, it was also very difficult to have so much unstructured time. At first I felt guilty that I did not have a job. Gradually, I discovered how much of a challenge it was to make plans for daily activities and the general care of household needs. This was the beginning of the most difficult phase of my recovery: facing the reality of disabilities created by the stroke and seeing the negative impact on day-to-day living. It was very difficult and frustrating.

Still, thanks to the therapists at Genesis and Mother Nature, I had a very good physical recovery and I could drive. That made it possible to do many household tasks as well as grocery shopping and running nearby errands. We lived in a place that had nearby access to grocery shopping, our bank, the post office, and a small public library. I was fortunate to be able to go to the library for a book, the post office, or the bank. While Jerry continued to feel concerned about my driving, it was a practical matter for me to take care of some errands while he was at work. That made me feel better and took some pressure off of Jerry as well.

Very slowly I began to discover that I could be more successful in my efforts if I simply wrote down what I wanted to get done the next day. I would start by making a list of tasks to be done. They were pretty simple: clean, go to the store, make dinner. Keeping up with grocery shopping could be tricky because I had to write down what to buy as soon as I knew what we wanted or needed. I realized that tasks did not seem to get done if I did not write them down. Over time things did get easier. The wall calendar became a vital element of my life. Some problems were not easy to anticipate.

One night after cooking dinner on my new smooth top range, we sat eating; and after a short time, Jerry noticed that the cook top burner light was on. I got up to see what was happening and discovered that I had not only left the burner on, but the Revere Ware pan was sitting there with the copper melting onto the cooktop. I quickly removed the pan and turned off the heat, but the residue on the cooktop would require some serious scrubbing. Jerry was unhappy and I was unhappy, but I assured him that I would be able to get it cleaned up. It turned out to be true that I could get it clean enough to use, and it did not have any debilitating damage. It had only slight residual discoloring. It was still a disturbing incident and one that I did not wish to repeat. This was not my first mistake with a burner. On a different occasion I left a burner on, then absently placed a glass casserole on the burner (thinking it was off). In the middle of dinner we heard a pop sound and found the dish broken on the cooktop. A different mess but not as bad as the copper pot bottom. "Well," Jerry said, "at least we were able to hear it." Still, I was very unhappy to be forgetful in this particular manner. It is definitely dangerous to walk away from the stove and leave a burner on.

My stamina continued to be a problem and would often interfere with my ability to complete housework or run errands or to simply remember my tasks for the day. Still, it got a little easier day-by-day to figure out the best method for getting things done. Eventually I decided that I was spending too much time without formal exercise. Since I still had my mountain bike from New Hampshire, I decided to see if I could start riding it around our neighborhood. Jerry agreed that it was a good idea and he wanted to try riding also. We took out the bikes and, after some minor struggle, I was able to get on the bike and peddle away. Jerry got on his bike too and we went around our block with success.

It felt good to be able to ride, even though it was tricky with my uncoordinated movements and my weak left side. It became obvious that riding a straight line was not too difficult, but making turns did present some trouble. I enjoyed my ride enough to be confident, so later I started to take short rides in our neighborhood early in the morning one or two times a week. This proved to be a good activity and took the place of my

3 times a week step aerobics. Since it was clear that step aerobics classes would not be possible, it was important to have some physical activity besides housework to help me improve and maintain my strength and stamina. It was important for me to continue to take care of household shopping and running errands so that Jerry would have some free time on weekends. This was a good thing. My physical abilities were improved enough that driving was not too strenuous for the short distances necessary for grocery shopping, the bank, or the post office. Unfortunately, my cognitive skills were a continuous challenge. This was all new to me. Shopping had always been a joint activity for us and it was odd to be taking on these things on my own. It was also strange not to go to work every day. I learned to be careful in making shopping lists and making sure to keep track of our needs. Over time it became easier and more enjoyable to take care of the little things like grocery shopping, the bank ,or the post office. During holidays I would do the family gift wrapping and mailings from the post office or the UPS store nearby.

Something that I did not think about causing trouble was residual noise in my ears after the seizures. It was only a minor thing, but on occasion it could be troublesome. One day in the middle of vacuuming, it happened that the phone rang and also someone was at the front door. I could easily distinguish the phone but the doorbell took me a little longer. Getting to the door, turning off the vacuum cleaner, and answering the phone was a bit of a struggle. Although it worked out well, it was a reminder that things were not so simple for me Nearly falling from tripping on the cord to the vacuum cleaner, then grabbing the phone, and rushing to the door was quite comical.

Other small things that gave me a feeling of discouragement showed up in ways I did not think about. My neighbor would often invite me to join her for lunch or dinner (if Jerry was out of town). Once we went to lunch at a nearby restaurant that we both enjoyed. I ordered the Salad Nicoise. This was served with the salad dressing in a small bowl alongside the salad. While eating I had not looked for the dressing (it was on the left). Suddenly, I discovered that I had allowed myself to rest my left hand near the plate and knocked the dressing onto my lap. "Well," my neighbor said, "at least it's on your napkin." We both got a good laugh out of it, but it was still a little disturbing. I had not previously taken much notice of my left side neglect problems, but it was clear that I needed to be doing that. This gave me pause in terms of driving since it is such a serious activity and requires full attention at all times. Knowing that neglect could be a problem for me was not comforting in the least.

There came a time when it was necessary to make decisions about my teaching certification. I had already decided against keeping my Florida Certified Behavior Analyst (CBA) certification. It was logical that my teaching certificate was unnecessary as well. Due to my cognitive disabilities, it was unrealistic to consider returning to teaching. At one point I had told my doctor that I recognized that if I worked for myself I'd get fired. That being the case, it was not realistic to imagine going back to work, not at the hospital, not to a school, not anywhere. I also decided to give up my Society for Cognitive Rehabilitation (SCR) membership. Giving up these certifications and memberships felt strange and a little demoralizing, but it was practical, given my cognitive deficits. It was no longer realistic for me to work in any of the areas where I had previously been successful. Considering all the jobs that had been easy to learn and the respect from fellow professionals and the various honors that I had enjoyed, this was a big disappointment. It was so foreign to me that I could not do any of those things. Housework and cooking were suddenly a challenge, where previously while working they had been easy. It seemed that while everything had been easy before, some were now difficult, and some were impossible. While this was a continuous source of discouragement, it was also a call for me to try harder. Nevertheless, it simply felt like things would never improve.

There were a few good things to think about. I was able to be safe at home alone and do some tasks as well. Because I had always wanted to grow herbs for cooking, Jerry set up a small garden in the side yard. I planted tomatoes, parsley, basil, and a few other things. I also grew broccoli at one point. Even in the Florida heat and the sandy soil of Ponte Vedra Beach it was a success. Since it was an ongoing task to keep up the plants, I often had the opportunity to observe the numerous birds that frequented the marsh behind our house. Knowing this, Jerry bought me a small digital camera for Christmas. After that, I found that photography was a lot of fun. I could work in the garden and take pictures too. This added activity helped to foster more improvement in cognitive skills since I had to learn something new and keep up with everything else at the same time. It wasn't always easy, but there was more good than bad.

One day Jerry said, "We should ride our bikes to the beach on Saturday." Thankfully, we were close enough to do that without riding on Highway A1A. Since that sounded good to me, I agreed. We set out on Saturday morning riding out of our neighborhood and through the next one. We eventually came to a place that required crossing a busy street. Jerry crossed the street first while I worked to get myself positioned to push off. Unfortunately, when I looked out at the street there seemed to be entirely too much traffic and it froze me in place. Jerry was calling and motioning for me to come over, but I couldn't make my feet move. Needless to say, this caused some concern on his part until he could get back across to see if he could help me. We decided to turn around and go home. It was discouraging as well as puzzling. After that riding the bike was not as interesting.

In spite of my many difficulties, we have been fortunate to continue traveling from time to time. In most cases, we have worked around my cognitive issues without much interference with our plans. There have been, on occasion, cognitive problems that were unpleasant. On a trip to California when we were in the Atlanta airport, we went to board the airport tram to our gate. When the doors opened, Jerry stepped into the car but let go of my hand in the process. When I looked at the gap between the platform and the tram car, my feet stopped. It was like crossing an intersection on my bike. I could not move. The doors suddenly closed and the tram moved off. Jerry, on the tram and me on the platform. Fortunately, I had my boarding pass so I located a nearby map, found the gate and made it in time to board our flight. This was a bit of a scare for us both, but we didn't let it stop us from having a good time. We knew that there was always a chance that problems might develop due to my cognitive disabilities, but we also knew that we could find solutions if it became necessary.

Traveling also made me see the value of having an organized method for keeping perpetually necessary travel items. Things that are often needed in a hotel room, but frequently unavailable could be put together and easily found when it was time for them to be used. That brought about the development of the "travel box." I keep it in the closet and have small travel items that I pick and choose from depending on the trip we may take. This has been very helpful in travel planning and easier hotel stays.

Eventually, we had to start thinking about what we would do when Jerry retired. When I was younger, and before the stroke, retirement was a faraway concept best left to consider when it was close. Jerry, on the other hand, has always been one to look forward. He had spent plenty of time thinking about the best way to retire. So while he was still working, he was looking at places that might be good for retirement as well as the many varied aspects of retirement from finances to living conditions. When he was getting closer to age 65, he shared with me what he had learned about a few places around the country as well as within Florida. We talked about our preferences for where we might like to be. Since I was already "retired," my thoughts went to the practical side of things. We spent a lot of time talking about various options and began to seriously look at visiting some places.

There was a good friend of Jerry's from his days in Minnesota who, with his wife, had a winter home in Florida. We accepted invitations to visit them and discovered that we liked the part of Florida (Ocala) where they chose to escape the cold of Minnesota winters. When Jerry discovered that a particular 55+ retirement community there had recently opened up, we took advantage of our visits to Ocala and looked into the community. We discovered that there were swimming pools, tennis courts, a golf course, and a multi-use path winding through the community. We also found the housing to be very attractive and very similar to what we had in Ponte Vedra Beach. The differences in what the community had to offer in terms of lifestyle were significant, and it was easy to see ourselves living there. We eventually put our house in Ponte Vedra

Beach up for sale and began the slow process of deciding which area of the new 55+community we might want to move into. We had looked at several options but when we saw the maintenance free neighborhood, we felt it would be best. It was very practical in terms of finances and in quality of life. We knew that it would always be a challenge to keep up a yard and house, so being able to pay for lawn care and external house upkeep in one monthly fee was very attractive. I had been through all the aggravation of dealing with lawn care companies and other household upkeep, so I knew it would make it easier and simpler to live in a place that had those things built into them.

It still came as a bit of a shock when our house sold since we had been living there for 20 years. Making the move proved to be the same challenge that any move can be, but the new house in a new community took the sting out of it. Still, the more difficult aspects of moving to a new town involved finding a doctor, dentist, eye care practitioner, and a hairdresser. We had been seeing the same family care doctor for 20 years and that made it difficult to think about a change. I had already changed my neurologist once when my Genesis doctor retired to Virginia to start a winery. I found a neurologist in Ocala but had to change again when they left their practice to teach at a Medical School. I finally found another neurologist in Ocala. From the beginning of the seizure problem, I had been assured that it would likely be a permanent problem and that medication would also be a permanent need. I had queried each neurologist on several occasions about the possibility of getting off the seizure medication with no success. Then on a routine visit my Ocala neurologist surprised me by recommending that I stop taking the seizure medication. I would not argue with that idea so he took out a note pad and wrote a taper schedule for me to follow.

The process would take 4 weeks using a gradual step down process to decrease and then discontinue the pills altogether. The biggest downside of the process was that I could not drive for the week before, and all during, and the week after the taper was complete. Although I did not enjoy this thought, it was more important to me to discontinue the medication. After the process was completed, the doctor ordered an EEG to check for seizure activity. After that he went over the results, telling me that there was no indication from the test of any activity in my brain to indicate any problem without medication. That was the best news he could have given me. Naturally, I would continue to see him in the future if I had any new problems.

We have been very happy to live in our small neighborhood for the past 10 years. We are able to do some traveling and enjoy local events as well. This is a very positive thing. Many of our friends agree that as long as possible we should do the things that we are able to do since none of us will be getting any younger. Although we have excellent experiences living here, every day presents a new set of challenges. The cognitive problems that have resulted from the stroke as well as the physical ones make every activity more difficult. I am slower at everything, and even simple tasks are harder than before. Historically speaking, I was always quick to learn things and once learned I tended to do very well. Cooking a complex meal could be quite easy for me. Now though, it is a struggle to get anything accomplished. Still, our surroundings are lovely, and we have many things to be happy about. I missed my garden at first, but our screened lanai works well for pots of herbs that can be used in cooking.

I am continually reminded of various problems created by my stroke. Although our community has both an indoor as well as an outdoor pool, I have been in neither one. I have lost my ability to enjoy swimming. Truthfully, I cannot claim to swim in any classic sense. I have often admitted that I do not know how to swim; I know how not to drown. As kids, my sisters and I did spend some time learning how to not drown in the Whiting Field Naval Base pool. In college there was a pool at the apartment complex where I lived and I did take advantage of it from time to time during the summer months. While we lived in Pensacola, Jerry and I enjoyed going to the beach regularly.

After my stroke I became somewhat claustrophobic. Pulling shirts over my head became bothersome. During pool therapy sessions, the therapist kindly did not require that I put my head under water. It was not necessary when using the special exercise equipment for the pool. It was unpleasant to find that getting under the shower made me uncomfortable too. This problem has improved, but has not gone completely away. The shower is not as unpleasant, but getting a shirt over my head still makes me uncomfortable. My left side continues to be less helpful than before, and that means overuse and ongoing pain for my right side. I continue as well to struggle with keeping memory strategies in use. I make lists or notes but I have to be careful. It can get confusing or overwhelming if there are too many lists or notes. Still, over time things have improved and continue to do so. I keep up my physical activity by walking every day as well as keeping up with basic housekeeping. I still cook regular meals and sometimes even go for a somewhat complicated recipe. I currently have 110 cookbooks that I have used over the years, so I am very thankful to be able to continue to put them to use. It is also possible to indulge in cooking with a culinary interest group within our community. I struggle with planning meals and executing the plans, but it is better than the early years immediately after my stroke.

All the while, I am constantly reminded about how very fortunate I am to be alive and be as active as I am. With all the limitations put on me by the stroke, it could be much worse. I see my blessings every day in the friends and neighbors around me and in the many things that I am able to do. Sometimes it isn't easy to think about the good things in life since the bad things are what get in our way. I know the difference between what I could do before the stroke and how the stroke changed me. Yet, I feel much better about my life than when I first lost my job as a cognitive therapist. I still find that I am susceptible to the "what if" and "if only" thoughts. In the end, however, it comes back to the facts. This is how things are; there is no way to know what might have been if my stroke had not happened. There is no reason for me to think about that. It can be very difficult to ignore the idea that you might have had a better life now if there had not been a stroke to interrupt/stop you.

There are people who have written excellent books about their stroke experience using the term "lucky" or "luck." These include Kirk Douglas who wrote **My Stroke of Luck**, Dr. Howard Rocket who wrote A **Stroke of Luck**, and Janet R. Douglas who wrote **A Wonderful Stroke**

of Luck. I have no feeling of "luck" with my stroke. I do happen to be lucky, but it has nothing to do with my stroke. It is instead in spite of my stroke. I have good friends and neighbors. Most importantly, I have Jerry. The things that I am able to do in spite of my stroke are what make my life good and worthwhile. It is always good to be busy rather than bored. Jerry and I make commitments to friends for activities that are enjoyable. One of the many things that we continue to enjoy is musical events, concerts, and musical plays at the theater. My ability to sit through a concert or play without bursting into tears has become possible. The lability issue, while not completely gone, has improved significantly. Many times on an early morning walk, seeing the sun rise over the golf course, I say to myself "Who'd a thunk it?" I look at the many people I pass and know that I am in a good place. We can get very busy here and events are always taking place. There is the Ocala Civic Theater, the symphony, and several high schools that put on plays and concerts. We often ask ourselves how we managed to get to the doctor, dentist, and optometrist back when we were working. The calendar is often full, so it seems odd that we could have had those same appointments and still managed a 40 hour week job. I often say, though, "Better busy than bored."

Still, this can be a bigger problem than before. Keeping track of all the different activities and appointments can be overwhelming at times. Making sure the calendar is always up to date can be difficult. Jerry is often in the position of keeping it up or constantly reminding me to put something on it that I will be doing. It can be very frustrating for him when I fail to keep up my appointments on the calendar or if I don't tell him what I have going on so that it can be noted on the correct date. Keeping the grocery list current can also pose a problem. Something that I would not think about being a problem is that I "look normal" to people. That is a problem because looking "normal" makes people think you are "normal." While it is good that people don't see the flaws that I know are there, it makes it difficult to account for any of my out of the ordinary "not quite right" behaviors.

On March 24, 2020 we "celebrated" the 25th anniversary of my stroke. Under normal circumstances we would probably pick a nice place to go out and eat. But we were in the middle of the COVID-19 pandemic so we stayed home. I made Macadamia nut crusted Mahi-Mahi (fish) with jasmine rice and fresh asparagus. To complete the meal we opened a bottle of Viognier from Veritas Winery in Virginia that we knew would perfectly compliment the food. This is the winery that my former neurologist, Dr. Andrew K. Hodson, started after he retired from his medical practice back in the early 2000's. Although it may seem like a strange thing to celebrate, it feels entirely appropriate to us. We can celebrate not having to go to the hospital and all the other things that were involved immediately after having my stroke. I can celebrate being free of those issues and many other things as well. I have been quite fortunate in not experiencing any new stroke problems or seizures. My health is relatively good and this is definitely celebration worthy. As time goes by my thoughts often turn to not just what happened but also how much has changed both positively and negatively. I think about the time I spent in the hospital and how lucky I was to be able to have my rehabilitation therapy at Genesis.

Recently I lamented to someone that I used to be good at crafts and sewing, she asked "What changed?" It is always difficult to articulate to someone exactly what has changed to make me less able than before. It isn't simply being older; there are retired tailors in our community who do quite well. While being older certainly is an aspect of my situation, the stroke affected my coordination as well as motor planning. Knowing what needs to be done and seeing how to do it are not on an equal footing. I used to be able to think like that, but it has become substantially reduced. I also have become less detail oriented than before. This can be a problem in many ways in my daily living. I remember once at work someone remarking that I could tell someone to go to Hell and make them think it was their idea. I wasn't sure about that but I do know that I was able to be very diplomatic at times. Now I just blurt things out without much thought and it can be very unhelpful.

Other problems involve being able to react quickly to instructions, requests, or questions from other people. This is most often a problem with Jerry. We don't always see things the same way. His general reaction to my slow response is to raise his voice because he can't tell if I've heard him. I do have a hearing problem. This in turn causes me to have a poor reaction rather than a good one. This is a source of friction that had not existed prior to my stroke. I am not quick to see an error on the computer screen or in other things. Jerry reads things quickly and can spot a problem much faster than I can. I have always teased him about being a "speed reader." I am not certain at times what happens in my brain when we get into a situation that makes him raise his voice. I think I'm in a state called "flooding," a condition that involves sensory or emotional overload causing an inability to think clearly and make sense of what is happening. This is similar to the door bell and phone ringing at the same time while the vacuum cleaner is running. Highly emotional situations can also promote flooding. Flooding is not uncommon in either traumatic brain injury or stroke. During therapy, I perceived that not everyone recognized some of my behaviors as being stroke related, but I have questions about my perceptions as well. It is possible that seeing things through the changes of stroke did not offer me the best viewpoint. When I returned to work, it did seem that people were looking at me from a "before stroke" view and either not seeing the reality or just hoping that I was not as damaged by my stroke. I have no doubt the rehabilitation therapy that I received at Genesis was incredibly good, and I feel it has made all the difference in my recovery.

It has taken me a very long time to put down these words to tell my story of stroke survival and my rehabilitation experience. Because COVID-19 has imposed limitations on our travel and social activities, it has been easier to devote more time to finishing my writing. I was once quite good at typing and could write a research paper in a short period of time. I recently went looking for some chapters from some earlier versions of this story and found a chapter that I started in 1997. It is now 2021 and I realize that I have written many chapter versions and made more than enough mistakes. I used to be fast with my fingers, but now things go slowly and at times haltingly. My profanity laced sessions of working on my story would be embarrassing if there was anyone to hear.

If Jerry is in the room he may ask me what I'm having trouble with, but he kindly ignores my swearing for the most part.

While my right hand retains agility and strength, my left is slow and stiff. Still, it is a start, stop, start, stop process as one thing or another interferes with progress. The noise in my head is never gone. It can be difficult to know if there is an actual noise, like the doorbell, or if it's just noise in my head. My left arm is heavy at times and my hand may press keys on the keyboard unknown to me so that strange screens pop up and hinder my progress. At the end of any amount of typing my right hand and arm are always sore and tired. I continue to struggle with emotional lability from time to time, but it is not as bad as it was in the past. In addition to all the physical issues, cognitive issues also came into play when dealing with word processing programs or with a new computer. Microsoft Word has been and will continue to be a challenge for me cognitively. These physical and cognitive issues were significant factors in the length of time it has taken to complete this book.

Yet, these problems are offset by the good things in my life. We still travel from time to time and we hope to reconnect with family and friends when the COVID pandemic subsides. I am always grateful for not only what I have, but also what I don't have. I have friends, activities, travel, books to read, music, and many other things to enjoy. I do not have a wheelchair or walker. Although I still have left side weakness, I do not have confinement of my limbs. I also do not have an inability for self-care, although I do have some minor difficulties. I still enjoy cooking and actually enjoy being able to clean my house. While cognitive challenges continue to be an issue, it is not as bad as it might be.

I can't recall ever being inspired to write creatively. When I was working on my Master's degree, I learned how to write research papers. Of course, that was back in 1986 and my first writing was done on Jerry's portable Osborne computer with a dot matrix printer. I was using WordStar at that time. Eventually, having to write so many papers made me buy a different computer for myself. I still had WordStar, but I got a Tandon computer using those big 5.25 floppy discs. Still, it got me through my Master's degree quite well. After settling in Ponte Vedra

Beach, we both moved on to different computers using the newer 3.50" floppy discs. That is the reason I felt somewhat comfortable starting to write this story. I did well in school, so it seemed like a natural thing for me to write. The difference is that if I'd wanted to write a book before my stroke it would have been relatively fast. Now, it takes forever to get anywhere. So after 25 years I'm still working to make it right. Writing papers is quite obviously not the same as writing a book. A paper is shorter and more precisely defined. A book has multiple parts. The benefit of my paper writing experience was in being able to think about the book logically and in a more or less linear fashion.

Although I have labored on the text myself, it has not been an entirely independent process. Jerry has aided and assisted me from the beginning. He has given me the benefit of his talents as an editor and as a sounding board. I could not do this on my own after my stroke. Before it was a very different story. I once wrote a paper for a class in a few hours. Jerry said, "I guess you wrote it in your head first." That did seem to be how it went back then. After the stroke what I have in my head is not easily put into print. Still, it does get there, very slowly but surely. It can be unsettling to know that I once worked as a cognitive rehabilitation therapist and actually knew what to do with or for someone who had a brain injury or stroke, but my stroke changed all that. I have found that knowing what to do is not quite as easy as it once was. What I have discovered is that some of the tried and true techniques of therapy, such as making lists or writing reminder notes, actually does work. Having social interactions and a variety of activities is also helpful for good mental health. I continue to struggle to control my thought processes during conversation. I am frequently reminding myself that just because something is in my head, it doesn't have to come out of my mouth. This can make for awkward situations. It is obvious, to me at least, that all of these techniques will be of immense importance as I age. Memory issues continue to cause me trouble and poor planning ability effects everything. Even my ability to cook can be negatively impacted by both memory and planning problems.

While it is obvious that I have been extremely fortunate in my recovery, it is unfortunate that very many problems remain. My physical abilities are good, but not like before. I recognize that I must continually learn to live with my limitations. I know that life may become more difficult as time goes by, but I choose to believe that I will be okay.

Author's Note

The events in this book are true. They are as accurate as I am able to recall and I tell them to you as well as I am able. I cannot guarantee that each detail is 100% accurate due to the long time since my employment as a cognitive rehabilitation therapist and my stroke. For any discrepancies or inaccuracies, I apologize. Things happened as I have described and are as accurate as my memory will permit. Over the years, I have struggled with a variety of technical difficulties related to the computer and word processing. For those problems, I have turned to Jerry for help. He has helped me navigate the different problems as they have occurred. I could not have done this alone.

Gratitude

I owe a debt of gratitude to many people at Genesis Rehabilitation Hospital: to Cynthia, Charles, Shirley, Rich, Travis, Allison, Kathy A., Kathy M., Alex, Julie, Russell, Deborah D., Jim, and Moira . I also thank the doctors: Murray, Ahn, and Hussain. Many thanks also to the nursing and aide staff as well. My sincere thanks to The PA's: Larry, Don and Sally. Finally, I must greatly thank the administration of Genesis Rehabilitation Hospital.

Also gratitude to my therapy team:

Alice, Ceil, Lisa, Inga, Gary, Dr. Woods, Dr. Hofmann, Dr. Hodson and all the nurses who gave me an excellent rehabilitation experience and made my recovery that much better. I have been extremely fortunate to know and work with these dedicated individuals. Thanks to my outpatient team, and Trish. Thanks to Dr. Crosson and Dr. Brott as well as my Ocala neurologist, Dr. Gaudier.

I thank my helpful neighbors in the Santa Fe neighborhood of Stone Creek, especially Kaye Abight and Bill Freeman for the generous gift of their time to read and edit my text. Also to Penny, Susan, and Joey who also read and offered advice. Special thanks to Madison for her expert editing and advice. I am truly fortunate to have these people in my life to offer assistance in my endeavor. Thanks also to my fellow Stone Creek authors: P.D. Egan (*The Girl on the Bridge*) and M. K. Bel Cher (*The Office Wife, Andrea's Story*), for their encouragement and support. I also thank my sister-in-law, Lynne Martin (*Home Sweet Anywhere*).

Most importantly, thanks to Jerry.

Resources

For Rehabilitation:

Brooks Rehabilitation Hospital:
   https://brooksrehab.org/

The Society for Cognitive Rehabilitation:
   https://www.societyforcognitiverehab.org/

For Stroke:

The American Stroke Association:
   www.heart.org

American Heart Association:
   www.heart.org

For Wine:

Veritas Vineyards and Winery:
   www.veritaswines.com

Suggested Reading

Bolt-Taylor, Jill, *My Stroke of Insight*, Penguin Books, 2009

Douglas, Kirk, *My Stroke of Luck*, Harper Collins, 2002

Douglas, Janet. R. OT, *A Wonderful Stroke of Luck,*
    Archway Publishing, 2018

Kamada, Laurel, *Transformed in a Stroke*, Toplight Books, 2021

Meyerson, Debra E., *Identity Theft, Recovering Ourselves After Stroke*,
    Andrews McMeel, 2019

McCrum, Robert, *My Year Off*, Broadway Books, 1999

Osborn, Claudia, L., *Over My Head*, Andrews McMeel, 1998

Rocket, Howard, *A Stroke of Luck*, Rehabilitation Institute of Toronto
    Foundation, 1998

Seal, Avrel, *With One Hand Tied Behind M y Brain*,
    Texas Christian University Press, 2020

Stone, Sharon, *The Beauty of Living Twice*, Knopf, 2021

Taylor, Tichina, *Walking Miracle: Memoir of a 19-Year-Old Stroke*,
    J Kenkade Publishing, 2019

Notes

Mary,

    I hope you enjoy
my story.

      Deborah and
Jerry

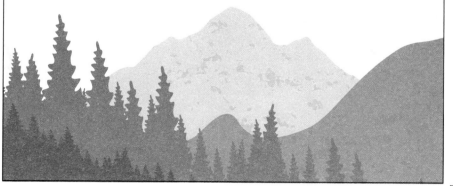

5

_____

_____

_____

_____

_____

_____

_____